LOCAL ANAESTHESIA IN DENTISTRY

DENTISTRY

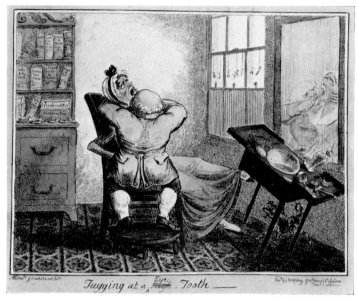

Past . . .

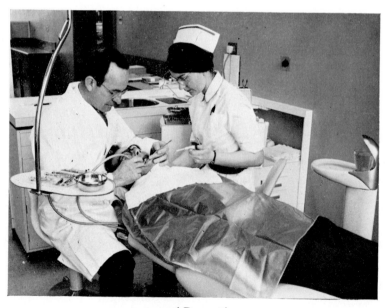

and Present!

A DENTAL PRACTITIONER HANDBOOK

SERIES EDITED BY DONALD D. DERRICK, D.D.S., L.D.S. R.C.S.

LOCAL ANAESTHESIA IN DENTISTRY

GEOFFREY L. HOWE

T.D., M.D.S. (Dunelm.), M.R.C.S. (Eng.), L.R.C.P. (Lond.),
F.D.S. R.C.S. (Eng.), F.F.D. R.C.S. (Irel.)

Professor of Oral Surgery and Oral Medicine,
University of Hong Kong
Formerly Professor of Oral Surgery,
Universities of Durham, Newcastle-upon-Tyne, and London

and

F. IVOR H. WHITEHEAD

F.D.S. R.C.S. (Eng.)

Consultant Dental Surgeon, Dudley Road Hospital, Birmingham
Honorary Senior Clinical Lecturer in Oral Surgery and Oral Medicine
University of Birmingham

SECOND EDITION

BRISTOL: JOHN WRIGHT & SONS LTD.

1981

Published by John Wright & Sons Ltd., 42–44 Triangle West, Bristol BS8 1EX.

First Edition	1972
Revised Reprint	1975
Second Reprint	1977
Second Edition	1981

British Library Cataloguing in Publication Data
Howe, Geoffrey L.
    Local anaesthesia in dentistry. – 2nd ed.
    – (A Dental practitioner handbook)
    1. Anesthesia in dentistry
    2. Local anesthesia
    I. Title   II. Whitehead, F. Ivor H.
    617′9676   RK510

ISBN 0 7236 0599 8

PRINTED IN GREAT BRITAIN BY
HENRY LING LTD., A SUBSIDIARY OF JOHN WRIGHT AND SONS LTD., BRISTOL,
AT THE DORSET PRESS, DORCHESTER

PREFACE

THE widespread use of local anaesthesia in many branches of dentistry makes it necessary for the dental undergraduate to acquire a working knowledge of this important subject fairly early in his career. In order to obtain clinical experience in other dental subjects, he often has to do this before he has studied pharmacology, medicine, or surgery in any depth.

Personal experience has led the authors to the conclusion that this objective is best achieved if the initial teaching is confined to basic principles and instruction in the use of well-tried and widely accepted techniques. In this way the student quickly acquires a basis for further study of the subject and a yardstick with which to evaluate the merits and demerits, advantages and disadvantages of other procedures.

In most dental schools local anaesthesia is taught by means of lectures, seminars, and clinical demonstration. This introductory text is designed to supplement and in no way replace these excellent methods of teaching. For the sake of clarity and continuity, discussions of controversial topics, references to the literature of the subject, and the description of more elaborate techniques which are rarely used have been omitted from the text. We hope that this book will help the student to acquire basic skills and encourage him to further study in this fascinating and important aspect of work in his chosen profession.

SECOND EDITION

As knowledge advances and opinions change even the simplest textbook must be updated if it is to continue to be of value. Despite its popularity to date, this little book is no exception to the rule and we have endeavoured to bring it up-to-date whilst carefully attempting to retain its character. Thus, whilst we have made a number of textual alterations and replaced many illustrations the format, style and size of the book remain unchanged.

It is a pleasure to acknowledge that we have been greatly helped by the constructive comments of many colleagues and friends, and we are indebted particularly to Mr. M. R. Sharland and his colleagues, University of Birmingham Dental School, for the new illustrations.

Hong Kong   G.L.H.
Birmingham   F.I.H.W.
1981

v

CONTENTS

CONTENTS

LOCAL ANAESTHESIA IN DENTISTRY

CHAPTER I

PAIN

Pain and pleasure are simple ideas incapable of definition.
Burke

A STUDY of contemporary records reveals that dentistry in the past was often a painful and even barbarous affair. Progress in the treatment of dental disease had to await the development of methods of pain control. The skilful use of such techniques has made painless dentistry a reality in recent years and the mastery of pain has proved to be an essential pre-requisite to the provision of a high standard of dental care.

Most patients seek dental treatment either for the relief of pain or in the hope of avoiding it at a later date. Pain may therefore be regarded as the *raison d'être* of the dental profession. Modern dental surgeons aim to cope with the ravages of dental disease as early as possible, before pain super-venes or the extraction of teeth is required. The main factors that delay the attainment of this objective are the patient's apathy, ignorance of dental matters, and the fear of pain. Whilst dental health education will of neces-sity take some time to combat apathy and ignorance, modern methods of pain control utilized in a skilful manner can do much to abolish the fear of pain in relation to dentistry. An understanding of the nature of pain is essential for those who aspire to manage it.

BASIC CONCEPTS

Although virtually everyone has experienced pain at some time and therefore from personal experience knows of its existence, no satisfactory definition of pain exists. Whilst it is often described in dictionaries as either a distressing sensation as of soreness, or as a disturbed sensation causing suffering or distress, these descriptions can apply equally well to other conditions. The difficulty arises because almost any stimulation carried to excess can result in pain. Furthermore, pain is almost always compounded with other sensations and attitudes, and reactions to it may be affected by both emotional and cultural factors.

To simplify matters it is convenient to divide pain into two components, perception of pain and reaction to pain.

Pain Perception.—The skin that covers the body and the mucous mem-branes that line some of its orifices are provided with numerous nerve-end organs for the perception of touch, temperature, and pain stimuli. The end organs which subserve pain are free non-medullated fibres and the application of an electrical, thermal, chemical, or mechanical stimulus to them may produce an impulse, or wave of excitation, in the nerve-fibres which is self-propagating and of uniform intensity. This is because each fibre obeys the 'all or none' law, that is to say, if a stimulus is sufficient to produce an impulse at all, the resultant impulse is of a uniform pattern and cannot be magnified by increasing the amount of the exciting stimulus. The severity of the pain perceived by the subject is governed by many factors one of which is the number of nerve-fibres that are activated and not by alterations in the size of the impulses conveyed by individual nerve-fibres.

The stimulus is conveyed along neural pathways to the thalamus, sharp pain being conducted by peripheral nerve-fibres with an axon core of larger diameter than those which convey dull pain.

Pain Reaction.—As the mechanism for pain perception works on the 'all or none' principle it is generally agreed that if a unit stimulus is applied to two individuals they should both perceive the same amount of pain. However, experience shows that in these circumstances whilst one individual may cry out and gesticulate wildly another seems to ignore the stimulus. The variable response to identical pain stimuli is not due to a difference in pain perception but to a variation in pain reaction. 'Pain reaction' is the term used to describe the integration and appreciation of pain within the central nervous system which occurs in the cortex and posterior thalamus. This is a variable factor which accounts for the clinical observation that the intensity of pain and the patient's response to it may vary not only between individuals but also from time to time in the same individual.

Pain Threshold.—This term is employed when the variable response to pain is being discussed. A patient is said to have a *high* pain threshold when he exhibits little or no reaction to a painful stimulus, whilst a patient with a *low* pain threshold is liable to react violently to an identical or even lesser stimulus. In other words, *pain threshold is inversely proportional to pain reaction.*

The pain threshold also varies between individuals and in the same individual at different times. Some factors which determine the level of tolerance include:—

1. *Psychological Make-up*.—Whilst it is readily apparent that emotionally unstable persons have a low pain threshold, it is easy to forget that each and every one of us is affected by our attitude towards the procedure, the operator, and our surroundings. In some patients previous painful experiences have visual or olfactory associations which may lower their pain threshold on subsequent occasions.

2. *Fear and Apprehension of Dental Treatment*.—Nervous patients become hyper-reactive and tend to magnify pain out of all proportion. It is therefore essential to attempt to secure the patient's confidence by all possible means and as early as possible (*see* page 31).

3. *Fatigue*.—As tiredness increases the pain threshold is lowered.

4. *Age*.—Whilst older patients usually tolerate pain well, children often have low pain thresholds and also find difficulty in distinguishing between pain and pressure.

The Anatomical Basis of Dental Pain

Impulses originating in the nerve-endings of the dental pulp and the supporting structures of the teeth are conveyed to the central nervous system by the second (maxillary) and the third (mandibular) divisions of the fifth cranial or trigeminal nerve (*Fig.* 1). From cell bodies in the Gasserian ganglion these neural pathways pass to the sensory nucleus of the trigeminal nerve which is situated in the medulla oblongata and extends to the level of the second cervical segment of the spinal cord. They then

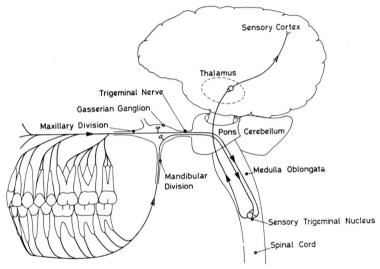

Fig. 1.—Sensory nerve supply of the teeth. The direction of impulses is indicated by the arrows.

pass via the trigeminal lemniscus to the postero-ventral nucleus of the thalamus and then via connecting neurones to the postero-central convolutions on the contra-lateral side of the cortex of the brain. Interruption of these neural pathways at any level may abolish the sensation of pain.

Current Views

Whilst knowledge of the anatomy and physiology of the nervous system is expanding constantly the precise mechanisms involved in the perception of pain have yet to be determined. The so-called Gate Control Theory (*Fig.* 2) has attracted considerable attention as a possible explanation of the manner in which pain impulses are modulated. According to this hypothesis, the passage of afferent pain impulses is either inhibited or facilitated in the substantia gelatinosa of the spinal cord or the caudal nucleus of the trigeminal nerve. It affords an explanation for the fact that at one and the same time impulses conveying differing sensations may be transmitted faithfully, modified, or delayed. The demonstration of the presence of pain-inhibiting substances such as endorphines in the central nervous system has lent support to this fascinating concept. It is believed that for pain to be experienced, cells transmitting via the anterior and/or lateral spinothalamic tracts must be activated. The Gate Control Theory postulates that an intermediary cell acts as a 'gate' to each transmitting cell and normally inhibits its activity. It is suggested that the activity of the intermediary cell is governed by the balance between the afferent impulses carried in the axons of the rapidly conducting thick myelinated A and B fibres and the more slowly conducting thin non-myelinated C fibres. The A and B fibres transmit impulses conveying common sensation and are inhibitory in this context, whilst the C fibres transmit impulses concerned with pain and diminish the inhibitory effect of the intermediary cell. It is suggested that the 'gate' is also influenced

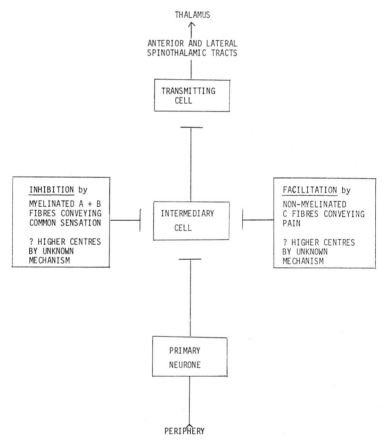

THALAMUS

ANTERIOR AND LATERAL
SPINOTHALAMIC TRACTS

TRANSMITTING
CELL

INHIBITION by

MYELINATED A + B
FIBRES CONVEYING
COMMON SENSATION

? HIGHER CENTRES
BY UNKNOWN
MECHANISM

INTERMEDIARY
CELL

FACILITATION by

NON-MYELINATED
C FIBRES CONVEYING
PAIN

? HIGHER CENTRES
BY UNKNOWN
MECHANISM

PRIMARY
NEURONE

PERIPHERY

Fig. 2.—Diagrammatic representation of the Gate Control Theory.

by descending fibres in the reticular activating system and that this may be the mechanism by which such alternative sensory inputs as counter-irritation or audio-analgesia diminish perceived pain. In such instances the 'gate' is held closed by impulses transmitted via the A and B fibres.

As has been stated earlier, the emotional make-up and the previous experiences of the individual concerned may greatly modify his or her reaction to a painful stimulus, but neither the manner in which, nor the level at which, this occurs in the central nervous system is known at present. Whilst it is possible that the memory of an earlier painful dental episode in a somewhat emotional individual could result in an opening of the 'gate' thus producing an exaggerated reaction to a comparatively mild stimulus, no mechanism is known by which such a change could be affected. Despite these reservations, the gate control theory provides an explanation for and helps an understanding of many of the varying phenomena associated with pain.

CHAPTER II

THE CONTROL OF PAIN

PAIN may be abolished by interrupting the neural pathways at various levels and by different means which can produce either permanent or temporary results. This book is mainly concerned with some of the methods employed to produce temporary impairment of sensation at lower levels of the anatomical pathways.

The nerve-endings subserving pain can be stimulated by mechanical, osmotic, thermal, and chemical stimuli. Pain usually ceases immediately if the stimulus that is exciting the nerve-endings is removed. The pain that may accompany dental treatment is often due to instrumentation. It is seldom practicable to remove such a mechanical stimulus and yet complete the treatment. In these circumstances, it is usually possible to employ a local anaesthetic agent either to reduce or abolish the excitability of nerve-endings or to block the pathways along which painful impulses are conveyed to the brain. This method of pain control is described as either local analgesia or local anaesthesia. However, the terms 'analgesia' and 'anaesthesia' are not synonymous for important differences exist between them. *Analgesia* is loss of pain sensation unaccompanied by loss of other forms of sensibility, whilst *anaesthesia* is loss of all forms of sensation including pain, touch, temperature, and pressure perception and may be accompanied by impairment of motor function. As a general rule, a larger dose of drug is required to obtain anaesthesia than to induce analgesia. If only a part of the body is affected the terms 'local analgesia' and 'local anaesthesia' are used. Local analgesia usually suffices when teeth are being conserved whilst local anaesthesia is preferred for extraction of teeth.

If the whole body is affected the terms 'general analgesia' and 'general anaesthesia' are employed. The pains of childbirth are often controlled by the induction of general analgesia (so-called relative analgesia) whilst general anaesthesia is employed for major surgery. The agents employed to induce general anaesthesia abolish pain reaction by depressing the activity of the brain and producing unconsciousness. Other drugs, such as aspirin, produce a state of general analgesia and seem to raise the pain threshold.

CHOOSING A METHOD OF PAIN CONTROL

Many dental procedures are painless, but, where necessary, dentistry may be performed with the benefit of either local or general anaesthesia and the dental surgeon must assess the indications and contra-indications of both before deciding which to use in a particular instance. On many occasions either method will suffice and in these circumstances the patient may be allowed to choose between them. However, if there is a positive contra-indication to the method of anaesthesia for which the patient has a preference, the dental surgeon should not be persuaded to use a technique which is not in the best interests of his patient, but should follow the dictates of his trained opinion and clinical experience.

Hurry is the enemy of good dental surgery and an ill-chosen form of anaesthesia is a common cause of undue haste. The dental surgeon must learn to estimate, with accuracy, the time required to complete each procedure if he is to choose a form of anaesthesia that provides adequate operating time for the completion of his task.

GENERAL ANAESTHESIA

A good anaesthetist can usually provide five to ten minutes operating time under general anaesthesia in the dental chair without the risk of anoxia or other complications. Although some exceptionally experienced and skilled anaesthetists are able to double this operating time, as a general rule the dental surgeon should not choose this form of anaesthesia for any procedure which may last for more than five minutes. Indeed if a surgical procedure under local anaesthesia is likely to last more than about thirty minutes, the best interests of the patient will often be served if the operation is performed under a general anaesthetic with endotracheal intubation. This may necessitate admission to hospital.

Very large and very obese patients are often unsuitable subjects for a general anaesthetic in the dental chair, especially those who regularly drink large quantities of alcohol. The co-operation of the patient greatly facilitates dental treatment. Unfortunately some patients are incapable of this co-operation for such reasons as fear, apprehension, extreme nervousness, hysteria, mental deficiency, or insanity. Young children below the age of reason find it impossible to distinguish between pressure and pain and so are liable to prove uncooperative if local anaesthesia is used for dental extractions. In some instances the judicious use of premedication may make the employment of local anaesthesia possible but in most instances it is easier to treat such patients if general anaesthesia is used. The induction of general anaesthesia in these cases may be difficult and may tax to the full both the skill and patience of the most experienced dental anaesthetist.

Systemic disease may be the deciding factor that influences the choice of anaesthesia. Any disease that impairs either respiratory efficiency or the airway is a contra-indication to general anaesthesia in the dental chair. Chronic bronchitis, bronchiectasis, emphysema, tuberculosis, asthma, and excessive smoking interfere with respiratory exchanges, whilst nasal obstruction, paralysis of the vocal cords, and space-occupying lesions of the neck may interfere with the patency of the airway. Any acute infection of the respiratory tract is an absolute contra-indication to general anaesthesia in the dental chair and in these cases local anaesthesia should be employed if dental treatment such as an extraction cannot be postponed. Acute infection in the floor of the mouth is a contra-indication to any form of anaesthesia as an out-patient. Oedema of the glottis and laryngeal obstruction may complicate general anaesthesia in such circumstances, whilst local anaesthesia is impracticable. Patients with these disorders should be admitted to hospital and any necessary surgery performed under endotracheal anaesthesia.

Whilst patients with chronic rheumatic heart disease usually tolerate both surgery and anaesthesia better than the middle-aged or elderly patient with either hypertensive or ischaemic heart disease, most patients with any form of cardio-vascular disease do not withstand anoxia or hypotension well, however temporary it may be. For this reason it is better to avoid the use of general anaesthesia in these cases whenever it is practicable to do so.

The patient's tolerance to exercise is the best guide to his ability to withstand both anaesthesia and dental treatment. The patient afflicted with severe heart disease should be admitted to hospital for any form of oral surgery, whatever form of anaesthesia is to be used.

Many anaesthetists prefer not to administer a general anaesthetic in the dental chair to a pregnant woman as they fear that they may be blamed if foetal damage, abortion, or miscarriage ensue.

Epileptics are usually good subjects for any form of anaesthesia provided that they have not omitted to take the anti-convulsant drugs to which they are accustomed. However, the use of methohexitone is contra-indicated for this group of patients.

Local Anaesthesia

The widespread and increasing popularity of local anaesthesia and analgesia in dentistry is a reflection of its efficacy, convenience, and the relatively few contra-indications to its use.

The techniques of local anaesthesia are easily mastered and the equipment required is limited in amount, economical, and easily transportable. The patency of the airway is not impaired and so the anaesthetic can be administered by the operator.

Another important advantage of local anaesthesia is that its use enables the patient to co-operate with the dentist to facilitate his own treatment. Usually preoperative preparation of the patient is not required when local anaesthesia is utilized and the patients can leave the surgery unescorted and often return to work after a local anaesthetic has been used. For these reasons local anaesthesia is widely employed for dental operations lasting up to three-quarters of an hour.

The most important contra-indication to local anaesthesia is the presence of acute infection at the site of operation. Injections of local anaesthetic solution into acutely inflamed areas spread the infection and seldom produce anaesthesia (page 72). It is sometimes possible to employ regional anaesthesia to obtain the desired effect, but no attempt should be made to use an inferior dental block in patients with infections involving the floor of the mouth or retromolar area.

Comparatively few systemic conditions contra-indicate the use of local anaesthesia in a general dental practice. The agents employed for this purpose have not been found to affect the foetus and pregnancy is not a contra-indication to their use. However, patients afflicted with certain rare haemorrhagic diseases such as haemophilia, Christmas disease, or von Willebrand's disease should not be treated under local anaesthesia due to the risk of bleeding at the injection site. Patients afflicted with such diseases have died after being given an inferior dental block injection for conservative treatment. The dangers associated with dental extractions in these patients make admission to hospital and full haematological cover imperative.

Whilst some authorities advise the omission of adrenaline from the local anaesthetic solutions administered to patients suffering from cardio-vascular disease, it is the opinion of the authors that the small amount of adrenaline administered for dental purposes is, in fact, beneficial. The use of such solutions ensures more certain, prolonged, and profound anaes-thesia and thus decreases the amount of adrenaline secreted by the patient himself in response to pain or fear. Nevertheless especial care should be exercised when administering inferior dental injections to avoid giving an intravascular injection. The careful use of an aspirating syringe minimizes this risk.

The vasoconstrictor contained in most local anaesthetic solutions assists haemostasis and provides a comparatively bloodless field of operation and this materially assists the dentist when he is performing surgery on his patient. However, on occasions vasoconstriction is undesirable. For example, since the vascularity of any bone that has been subjected to therapeutic irradiation is impaired, further restriction of the blood supply due to the use of local anaesthetic solutions containing vasoconstrictors is to be avoided. It is preferable to perform oral surgery for such patients under general anaesthesia or if this is not practicable with a 'plain' local anaesthetic solution (*Table I*, page 14). There is, of course, no reason why such solutions cannot be used when conservation treatment alone is to be undertaken for patients who have had radiotherapy to the jaws.

Some patients acquire a sensitivity to certain local anaesthetic agents. Fortunately this abnormal reaction is specific to such a degree as to make it possible to utilize an alternative agent of a different chemical structure when a patient either gives a history of or exhibits sensitivity to a particular drug (page 82).

The many contra-indications, advantages, and disadvantages of local and general anaesthesia in the dental chair have been emphasized because of their importance. However, it must be remembered that both forms of anaesthesia have been in widespread use for a long time and that the mor-bidity is infinitesimal if care is taken in the selection of the appropriate method. The dental surgeon should always make careful inquiries into the general medical history of any patient consulting him and in cases of diffi-culty he should enlist the aid of the patient's physician before selecting the form of anaesthesia to be employed. As a general rule any patient classified as a poor anaesthetic risk is better treated as an in-patient under either local anaesthesia or endotracheal anaesthesia.

Types of Local Anaesthesia.—Local anaesthesia may be induced by interrupting the sensory nerve-supply at differing anatomical levels. Some of these sites are illustrated diagrammatically in *Fig. 3*.

If certain local anaesthetic agents, such as cocaine and lignocaine, are applied to the intact mucous membrane they pass through the epidermis and anaesthetize the nerve-endings. This technique is described as *topical*

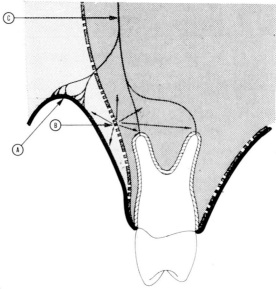

Fig. 3.—An anaesthetic agent deposited at different sites will produce different types of local anaesthesia. (*See text for explanation.*)

or *surface anaesthesia* (*Fig.* 3A) and is discussed on page 38. More commonly pain perception is abolished by depositing the anaesthetic solution around nerve filaments, a method called *infiltration anaesthesia* (*Fig.* 3B), which is discussed on page 40. A region of the body may be rendered anaesthetic by blocking conduction in the nerve-trunk supplying the area and this technique is known as *regional or block anaesthesia* (*Fig.* 3C) (page 45). Whilst it is possible to inject nerve divisions and ganglia these procedures are usually only employed by neurologists, when called upon to treat patients suffering from facial neuralgia, and have no place in routine dentistry.

CHAPTER III

THE DEVELOPMENT OF LOCAL ANAESTHESIA
IN DENTISTRY

LOCAL anaesthesia as it is known today began with the development of
the hypodermic syringe. Early types of this instrument were designed for
the subcutaneous deposition of drugs in fluid form. Credit for the proto-
type appears to belong to A. Neuner, of Austria, who introduced fluids
from a syringe into the eyes of animals via a hollow needle in 1827. The
first record of the application of such a principle in humans is attributed
to Zophar Jayne, of America, who in 1841 introduced a needle into a
patient through an incision in the skin.

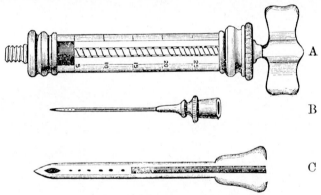

A.—Hypodermic syringe, as made for author.
B.—One of the gold tubular perforating needles.
C.—Enlarged view of B.

Fig. 4.—The illustration of Charles Hunter's syringe and needle as it
appeared in his book published in 1865.

In 1844 Francis Rynd, of Dublin, introduced a mixture of acetate of
morphine dissolved in creosote through skin incisions into the region of
the supra-orbital nerve for the treatment of trigeminal neuralgia. The
instrument used incorporated a spring-loaded device and utilized a trocar
and cannula through which the solution passed by gravity into the tissues.
Although it was displayed at the Great Exhibition in 1851, its description
was not published until ten years later. In 1858 Alexander Wood, of
Edinburgh, described his modification of a glass syringe with a piston and
piston-rod and a needle with a bevelled point. He stated that he had used
this instrument for the subcutaneous injection of muriate of morphia in
the treatment of neuralgia since 1853. This would appear to be the earliest
form of hypodermic injection in the modern sense. 1853 was also the year

in which Charles-Gabriel Pravaz, a French veterinary surgeon, reported the use of a syringe for introducing sclerosing solutions into the blood-vessels of animals. For this purpose he employed an all-metal syringe that incorporated a piston, piston-rod, trocar, and cannula.

Charles Hunter, in his book entitled *On the Speedy Relief of Pain and Other Nervous Affections by means of the Hypodermic Method*, that was published in 1865, claimed to have introduced the word 'hypodermic' six years earlier. He also recognized the systemic effects of drugs introduced by this route, whereas Wood had been concerned with their local action only. *Fig.* 4 illustrates the syringe that Hunter employed. Part of his description of this instrument reads as follows: 'The barrel is of glass with silver fittings and contains a piston which works by a screw-rod, each half turn of which expels half a minim . . .'.

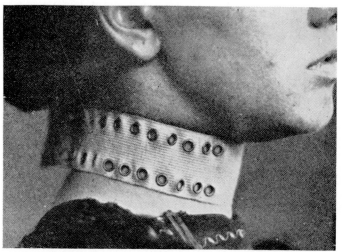

Fig. 5.—The illustration of a 'stasis bandage' from Fischer's textbook published in 1912.

In a textbook published in 1912 the possible systemic effects of local anaesthetic solutions were emphasized by Guido Fischer, a German, who advocated that a stasis bandage (*Fig.* 5) be fitted round the patient's neck. The purpose of this manœuvre was described as follows: 'This bandage produces stasis of the carotid arteries thus rendering cerebral anaemia less likely to occur, retaining the anaesthetic in the desired field for a longer period and still further retarding absorption.' Not surprisingly this technique has not found widespread acceptance!

The discovery of cocaine was a milestone in the development of local anaesthesia. Leaves of a plant called *Erythroxylon coca* were brought to Europe from Peru and in 1855 an alkaloid was extracted from them by F. Gaedcke, a French chemist. In 1860 Albert Niemann isolated the alka-loid in its pure form and named it 'cocaine'. Several studies on the pharmacology of cocaine were published but little of any practical value emerged. In 1884 the drug engaged the attention of Sigmund Freud, and it was he who encouraged Carl Koller to explore its possibilities. Koller, who was studying ophthalmology in Vienna, discovered that a solution of cocaine produced effective surface anaesthesia of the cornea.

Cocaine was soon tested elsewhere in the body as a surface anaesthetic and in the same year as Koller's work was published, William Steward Halsted, in America, used a solution of cocaine to produce anaesthesia of the inferior dental nerve. He subsequently became a victim of the drug's addictive properties, and took over two years to break himself of the habit.

The first record of the use of cocaine by injection in Britain appeared in the *Journal of the British Dental Association* in 1886, when William Alfred Hunt, of Yeovil, described its use in infiltration techniques.

In 1901 E. Mayer suggested the addition of a small quantity of adrenaline to the solution to promote vasoconstriction, prolong the duration, and intensify the depth of anaesthesia. Since both drugs were derived from natural sources, great variation occurred in their quality and efficacy. This stimulated efforts to produce them in the laboratory and success came in 1904. In this year A. Stolz prepared adrenaline in pure form and commercial quantities from animal tissues and Carl Theodor Liebermann and Friedrick Oscar Giesel prepared cocaine synthetically.

In 1905 Alfred Einhorn and E. Uhlfelder, two Swedish chemists, completed a long research project in which they discovered that the complete molecule of cocaine was not necessary for the production of local anaesthesia. They produced, synthetically, procaine hydrochloride which was tested clinically by Henrich Braun and marketed as 'Novocaine'. This substance was shown to be non-addictive and far less toxic than cocaine, capable of sterilization by boiling, and much less irritant to the tissues at the site of injection. For these reasons procaine quickly supplanted cocaine and is still used in some areas of medical and dental practice today. Procaine, with or without adrenaline, was initially only available in tablets that were dissolved in the appropriate quantity of sterile water by the dental surgeon.

Metal or metal and glass syringes with hypodermic needles were used to introduce the solution and in 1897 Freienstein, a German, invented the dental interchangeable needle. During the 1914–18 war Dr. Harvey S. Cook conceived the idea of the anaesthetic cartridge, the cartridge syringe, and double-ended needle (*Figs.* 9, 10, pages 22 and 23), and these became available in 1921. Later Ringer's solution was used instead of sterile water in order to produce an isotonic solution, and buffering agents were included in the early 1930s.

Slight variations in the procaine molecule have produced other anaesthetic agents and some of these are in use currently. A major rival, however, was discovered in 1943 when N. Lofgren, in Sweden, synthesized the anilide which was named 'Lignocaine' but is known as 'Lidocaine' in some countries. This anaesthetic agent was introduced into clinical practice in 1946 and is now the most widely used in the world. Research, however, continued and in 1956 mepivacaine came into clinical use to be followed in 1959 by prilocaine. These drugs are related chemically to lignocaine, the former being an acyl variant and the latter a toluene variant. They provide effective alternatives to lignocaine in clinical practice.

Table I.—Some Local Anaesthetic Solutions Available in Great Britain

N.B. Other solutions are available which contain differing strengths of these local anaesthetic agents either with or without one of the vasoconstrictors, the concentration of which may vary.

Approved Name of Anaesthetic Agent	Proprietary Name of Solution	Chemical Description of Anaesthetic Agent	Strength of Agent (per cent)	Vasoconstrictor	Concentration of Vasoconstrictor
Ester Linkage Agents Procaine	Novocain	Para-amino benzoate hydrochloride			1 : 50,000
Amide Linkage Agents Lignocaine	Xylocaine Xylotox Lidothesin Nurocain Lignostab A Xylonor Lignospan	Xylidide	2	Adrenaline	1 : 80,000
	Pensacaine				
	Scandonest Lignostab N Lidocaton Neo-Lidocaton				1 : 80,000 or 1 : 100,000
					1 : 100,000
	Xylotox Xylotox Plain Scandonest Plain		4	Nor-adrenaline	1 : 80,000
Prilocaine	Citanest 30	Toluene variant of xylidide	3	Nil	
	Citanest		3	Adrenaline	1 : 300,000
	Citanest Plain		3	Felypressin	0·03 I.U./ml
			4	Nil	—
Mepivacaine	Carbocaine Plain	Acyl variant of xylidide	3	Nil	—
	Carbocaine		2	Adrenaline	1 : 80,000

The synthetic local anaesthetic agents available at the present time thus fall into two major groups:—

1. Those which contain an ester linkage, e.g., procaine—

$$H_2N-\langle\bigcirc\rangle-CO-O-CH_2-CH_2-N\begin{smallmatrix}C_2H_5\\ \\C_2H_5\end{smallmatrix}$$

2. Those which contain an amide linkage, e.g., lignocaine—

$$\overset{CH_3}{\underset{CH_3}{\langle\bigcirc\rangle}}-NH-CO-CH_2-N\begin{smallmatrix}C_2H_5\\ \\C_2H_5\end{smallmatrix}$$

Slight modifications of these basic formulae have enabled pharmaceutical firms to market solutions under a variety of proprietary names. The proprietary names are related to the approved names in *Table I*, which is by no means comprehensive as other preparations are available. Due to reduced demand procaine is no longer available packaged in cartridge form. It has a continuing, though limited, application in other fields of medical practice. All other solutions detailed in *Table I* are available in cartridges. In most of the solutions listed, variations in the strength of the anaesthetic agent are related to differing concentrations of the vasoconstrictor agent. For example, when felypressin is omitted from Citanest with Octapressin the strength of the agent is increased to 4 per cent and this solution is marketed as Citanest Plain.

CHAPTER IV

LOCAL ANAESTHETIC SOLUTIONS

THE properties of some of the local anaesthetic solutions in use in dentistry at the present time are detailed in *Table II*. In general terms each of these preparations contains the following constituents: (A) A local anaesthetic agent. (B) A vasoconstrictor. (C) A reducing agent. (D) A preservative. (E) A fungicide. (F) The vehicle.

LOCAL ANAESTHETIC AGENTS

Despite the constant development of new drugs the ideal local anaesthetic agent has yet to be introduced into clinical practice. However, it is useful to consider the requirements of the 'ideal agent' when assessing the properties of the drugs used in dentistry.

1. Potency and Reliability.—The first requirement of such a substance is that when administered correctly and in adequate dosage it consistently produces effective local anaesthesia. Earlier agents (e.g., cocaine) were obtained from natural sources and there was considerable variation in their purity, potency, and reliability. These problems have been overcome by present-day methods of production and packaging. Thus experience has shown that approximately 98 per cent of injections using a 2 per cent lignocaine with 1:80,000 adrenaline solution are followed by effective anaesthesia.

A similar proportion of successful injections should be achieved with the other solutions listed in *Table II*.

2. Reversibility of Action.—The action of any drugs used to obtain local anaesthesia must be completely reversible within a predictable time. This requirement limits the number of agents that are acceptable for clinical use, although a number of other drugs (e.g., phenol and alcohol) have local anaesthetic properties.

3. Safety.—All local anaesthetic agents must have a wide margin of safety from the poisonous side-effects which are collectively known as 'toxicity'. This margin of safety is conveniently described as the therapeutic ratio which is expressed as:—

$$\frac{\text{Lethal Dose} \quad (LD_{50}) = \text{Dose which kills 50 per cent of a group of experimental animals}}{\text{Effective Dose } (ED_{50}) = \text{Dose which produces the desired effect in 50 per cent of a group of experimental animals}}$$

The higher the value of this ratio the greater the safety margin. Procaine has the highest therapeutic ratio, followed in descending order by mepivacaine, prilocaine, and lignocaine. The official maximum safe doses of these

Table II.—Comparative Values for Local Anaesthetic Solutions Available in Great Britain

N.B. All figures are approximate

Approved Name of Anaesthetic Agent		Procaine 2 per cent	Lignocaine 2 per cent	Prilocaine 3 per cent Citanest		Mepivacaine 3 per cent
				With 1:300,000 Adrenaline	With Octapressin 0·03 I.U./ml.	
Proprietary Name of Solution		Novocain with Adrenaline 1:50,000	Various (*See Table I*) with Adrenaline 1:80,000			Carbocaine
Recommended Maximum Adult Dosage	With vaso-constrictor	500 mg.	500 mg.	600 mg.	600 mg.	—
	Without vaso-constrictor	200 mg.	200 mg.	400 mg.	400 mg.	400 mg.
Surface Anaesthetic Properties		Minimal	Good	Slight		Minimal
Onset Time	Infiltration	3½ min.	1½ min.	1½ min.	1½ min.	2½ min.
	Regional	7¼ min.	4 min.	4 min.	4 min.	4½ min.
Duration of Soft Tissue Anaesthesia	Infiltration	2¼ hr.	3 hr.	2 hr.	2¾ hr.	1 hr.
	Regional	2¼ hr.	3 hr.	3 hr.	3½ hr.	2 hr.
pH Value	With vaso-constrictor	4	4	3·5	4·5	—
	Without vaso-constrictor	5·5	6	6		6·4

agents are modified by the addition of vasoconstrictors and are detailed in *Table II*. The toxic effect of these drugs is also increased by inadvertent intravascular injection (page 73).

4. Lack of Irritation.—No injury to or irritation of the tissues should result from the injection of a local anaesthetic agent. For this reason local anaesthetic solutions should be isotonic and have a *p*H compatible with that of the tissues.

5. Rapidity of Onset.—Ideally the injection of such an agent should be followed immediately by the onset of local anaesthesia. In this context it is important to appreciate the difference between the onset of 'changed sensation' which heralds analgesia and actual surgical anaesthesia with complete blockage of impulses. Experiments have shown that the mean onset time following infiltration anaesthesia using a 2 per cent lignocaine, 1 : 80,000 adrenaline solution is about 1 minute 20 seconds.

6. Duration of Effect.—In theory recovery of sensation should coincide with the completion of treatment. In practice the duration of anaesthesia is usually longer than is required for dental procedures.

The inclusion of a vasoconstrictor in a local anaesthetic solution affects the duration of anaesthesia and is discussed below. Lignocaine solutions produce the longest duration of anaesthesia, followed in descending order by those containing prilocaine, procaine and mepivacaine. The average duration of anaesthesia produced by the various proprietary preparations is shown in *Table II*.

7. Sterility.—Since local anaesthetic agents are introduced into the tissues it must be possible to sterilize them without affecting either their structure or properties. The dental surgeon can avoid this problem by using the products of reputable manufacturers, who use approved methods of sterilization such as ultra-filtration.

8. Adequate 'Shelf Life'.—Unless the local anaesthetic agent is stable in solution and compatible with the other constituents the 'shelf life' of the preparation will be reduced (*see below*, Vasoconstrictors). Most present-day solutions have a 'shelf life' of 2–2½ years, but unfortunately some manufacturers do not reveal either the date of manufacture or provide an expiry date for their products.

9. Penetration of Mucous Membrane.—Ideally the drug should have the property of penetrating mucous membrane so that topical anaesthesia is practicable. Lignocaine has this desirable quality whilst other agents possess it to an extent insufficient for clinical use.

VASOCONSTRICTORS

The addition of a small quantity of a vasoconstricting drug to local anaesthetic solutions has the following advantages:—

1. It reduces toxic effects by retarding the absorption of the constituents.

2. By confining the anaesthetic agent to a localized area it increases the depth and duration of anaesthesia.

3. It produces a relatively bloodless field of operation for surgical procedures.

The vasoconstrictors in general use are:—

1. Adrenaline (epinephrine), a synthetic alkaloid almost identical with the natural secretion of the adrenal medulla.

2. Noradrenaline (laevoarterenol, norepinephrine), a synthetic substance similar to the pressor amine secreted in the human body by monoaminergic neurons in the brain and at the adeno-neural and myo-neural junctions of the sympathetic nervous system.

3. Felypressin (Octapressin), a synthetically produced polypeptide similar to that secreted from the human posterior pituitary gland.

Both the depth and duration of anaesthesia may be modified by the amount of vasoconstrictor in the solution. For these reasons some manufacturers offer lignocaine solutions containing adrenaline or noradrenaline in concentrations of 1:50,000, 1:80,000, or 1:100,000. In general the lower the concentration of vasoconstrictor the less the depth and duration of anaesthesia.

Felypressin is only available in Citanest in a concentration of 0·03 I.U./ml.

The possible adverse effects of vasoconstrictors are discussed on page 9.

OTHER CONSTITUENTS

Reducing Agent.—Vasoconstrictors are unstable in solution and may oxidize, especially on prolonged exposure to sunlight. This results in the solution turning brown and this discoloration is an indication that such a solution must be discarded. In an attempt to overcome the problem a small quantity of sodium meta-bisulphite, which competes for the available oxygen, is included in the solution. Since this substance is more readily oxidized than adrenaline or noradrenaline it protects their stability.

Preservative.—Modern local anaesthetic solutions are very stable and often have a 'shelf-life' of two years or more. Their sterility is maintained by the inclusion of a small amount of a preservative such as caprylhydrocuprienotoxin which is included in Xylotox. Some preservatives, such as methylparaben, have been shown to produce allergic reactions in sensitized subjects (page 82).

Fungicide.—In the past some solutions tended to become cloudy due to the proliferation of minute fungae. In several modern solutions a small quantity of thymol is added to serve as a fungicide and prevent this occurrence.

The Vehicle.—The anaesthetic agent and the additives referred to above are dissolved in modified Ringer's solution. This isotonic vehicle minimizes discomfort during injection.

METABOLISM AND EXCRETION

The detoxification of local anaesthetic agents differs according to their chemical structure.

The ester type agents are dissociated by esterases in the blood and liver and hydrolysed to benzoic acids and alcohol. Some oxidation may also take place in the liver and all breakdown products are excreted in the urine.

The metabolism of the amide type agents is more complex and somewhat slower. It appears that breakdown does not occur in the blood-stream and that hydrolysis takes place mainly in the presence of catalysts in the liver. The products are then oxidized further and some conjugation with glucuronic acid takes place. Finally, conjugated and unconjugated products are excreted in the urine.

Patients afflicted with impaired liver or renal function should not be given large doses of local anaesthetic agents due to the risk that failure of metabolism and excretion may result in over-dosage.

MODE OF ACTION

All anaesthetic agents are formed by the combination of a weak base and a strong acid. They are readily hydrolysed in the alkalinity of the human tissues (pH 7·4 approx.) to liberate the alkaloid base which is then free to be taken up by the lipids in the nerve-fibre.

Since the hydrochloride salt is the most common form in which the local anaesthetic agents are used, this process may be represented by the equation:—

$$\underset{\substack{\text{(anaesthetic}\\\text{salt)}}}{\text{B.HCl}} + \text{NaHCO}_3 \xrightarrow{pH\ 7·4} \underset{\text{(free base)}}{\text{B.}} + \text{NaCl} + \text{H}_2\text{CO}_3$$

The precise mode of action of the free base is not understood but there is a considerable amount of evidence that it prevents the increase in sodium permeability of the nerve membrane. The probable mechanism is illustrated in *Fig.* 6.

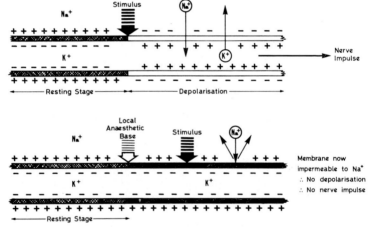

Fig. 6.—Probable mode of action of a local anaesthetic agent.
Above: In a normal afferent nerve-fibre an effective stimulus will cause depolarization and give rise to an impulse.
Below: When the axonal limiting membrane has been stabilized by a local anaesthetic agent depolarization is prevented and no impulse is conducted.

The type and size of the nerve concerned affect the rapidity of anaesthesia. A greater amount of solution and more time are required to anaesthetize myelinated nerves because the axon can only be affected by the anaesthetic agent at the nodes of Ranvier. Small nerve-fibres, such as those subserving pain and temperature, are anaesthetized more quickly than the larger motor and proprioceptive fibres.

CHAPTER V

EQUIPMENT

THE range of equipment available for the administration of local anaesthetics has been developed as a result of the need for convenience in use and the maintenance of sterility.

Many diseases are caused by infection with micro-organisms, and those micro-organisms that cause disease are described as being 'pathogenic'. If pathogenic micro-organisms are introduced into an injection site there is a serious risk that a local or systemic infection may result. The dentist must attempt to prevent the occurrence of this undesirable complication by sterilizing both the equipment and the materials being employed. *Sterilization* may be defined as the removal of all micro-organisms from a given object, or their effective destruction.

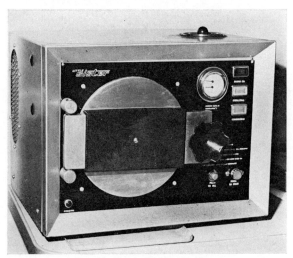

Fig. 7.—'Little Sister' autoclave.

In order to kill the most resistant micro-organisms, namely bacterial spores, it is necessary to subject them either to moist heat at 120° C. for 10–12 minutes in an autoclave (*Fig.* 7) or steam pressure sterilizer, or to dry heat at 160° C. for 60 minutes in a hot-air oven (*Fig.* 8). Water boils at 100° C. at normal temperature and pressure and bacterial spores may resist these conditions for 60 minutes, and fungi and thread organisms for 20 minutes. Therefore hot water 'sterilization' cannot produce sterility and as this form of disinfection is still widely employed in general dental practice it is fortunate that the majority of pathogenic bacteria that may be present are in the vegetative phase and are destroyed by immersion in boiling water for 5–10 minutes.

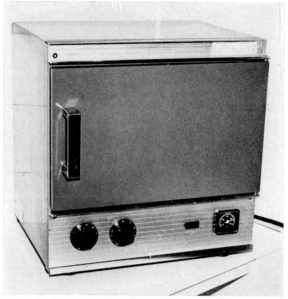

Fig. 8.—Electrolux 'Helios' dry heat sterilizer.

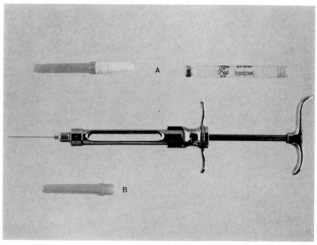

Fig. 9.—Cartridge syringe fitted with (A) disposable needle in its sealed plastic container and standard 2 ml. cartridge of solution. B, Detached needle guard.

SYRINGES

The most widely used local anaesthetic equipment in present-day dental practice is illustrated in *Fig.* 9. This basic design of syringe has been available for many years and alternative patterns have only been introduced in comparatively recent times. The syringe consists of a metal barrel and plunger united by a spring-loaded hinge mechanism. A double-ended needle is attached by means of a screw hub to the other end of the barrel. Opening of the hinge mechanism permits the insertion of a glass cartridge containing the sterile local anaesthetic solution (*Fig.* 10).

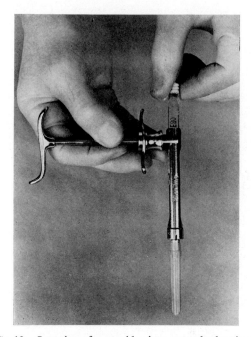

Fig. 10.—Insertion of a cartridge into a standard syringe.

Before the introduction into dental practice of effective means of sterilization it was only possible to disinfect a syringe and needle before use. In these circumstances the pre-sterilized contents of a cartridge could be contaminated whilst passing through the lumen of a non-sterile needle. This risk has been minimized by the introduction of pre-sterilized stainless-steel needles (page 26) although it is still possible for contamination to occur if the hub attachment of the syringe has only been disinfected. The other major short-coming of the assembly is that it does not permit the dental surgeon to aspirate prior to injection in an attempt to avoid depositing the solution in a blood-vessel. Accidental intravascular injection predisposes either to over-dosage effects or to interaction with other drugs that the patient may be taking.

The manœuvre of aspiration consists of withdrawal of the rubber plunger to create a negative pressure within the cartridge and is employed in order to ensure that a blood vessel has not been entered by the needle tip during its insertion into the soft tissues and prior to the injection of the solution. Positive aspiration results in a fine spiral of blood being clearly visible in the solution within the cartridge (*Fig.* 11).

A slight amount of aspiration may be achieved with a standard cartridge by making a small initial injection of solution and then releasing the pressure on the rubber plunger which then rebounds to produce an aspiration effect.

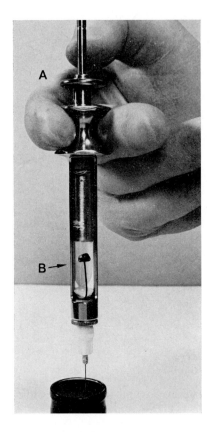

Fig. 11.—A Canadian aspirating syringe fitted with a disposable needle and loaded with a 1·8 ml. cartridge of solution. Ink has been used in this photograph to illustrate how the release of pressure with the thumb on the diaphragm (A) results in aspiration into the anaesthetic solution of a spiral of ink (B). (*Courtesy of Professor A. G. Parnell.*)

This crude procedure has been refined in the Astra aspirating syringe and cartridge. The open-sided aluminium alloy syringe is shown in *Fig.* 12A ready for use. The mechanism for achieving aspiration is illustrated in *Fig.* 12B in which it will be seen that it consists of a tapered socket within the rubber plunger into which the end of the metal piston fits. The manner in which aspiration is effected is shown diagrammatically in *Fig.* 13. Following placing of the piston end into the specially adapted plunger (A), slight pressure on the piston produces a bulge in the rubber plunger (B) which in turn exerts pressure on the solution in the cartridge. Release of this pressure produces suction (C). If the needle tip is in a blood-vessel, a thin spiral of blood which rapidly diffuses, will be seen in the solution (*Fig.* 11).

Other types of aspirating syringe are available, two of which are illustrated in *Figs.* 14 and 15. These rely upon a device at the end of the piston which is capable of engaging the rubber plunger to enable it to be withdrawn slightly up the cartridge after the initial injection. By this means an aspiration effect is produced. Since the movement required is best achieved by backward pressure with the thumb, many such syringes are manufactured with a ring-type of handle to facilitate this.

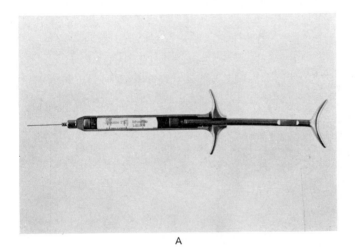

A

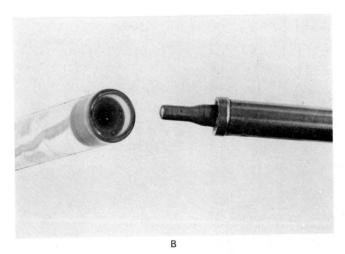

B

Fig. 12.—A, Astra aspirating syringe assembled ready for use. B, *See text for description.*

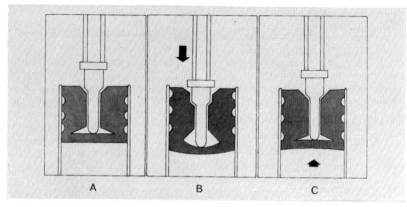

Fig. 13.—Mechanism of aspiration of Astra aspirating syringe. (*See text for explanation.*)

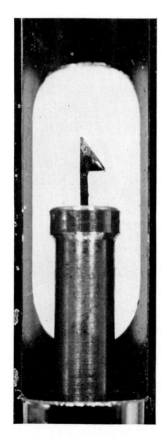

Fig. 14.—This harpoon-ended plunger rod is designed to pierce and hold the rubber plunger of the cartridge, thus permitting it to be withdrawn in order to produce aspiration.

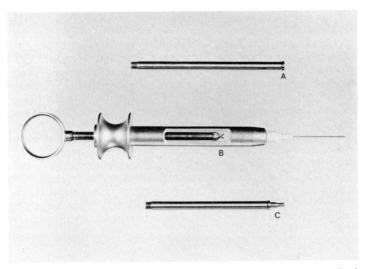

Fig. 15.—Ash syringe. Note interchangeable pistons:—**A**, non-aspirating; **B**, Spiral claw aspirating; **C**, Astra type aspirating.

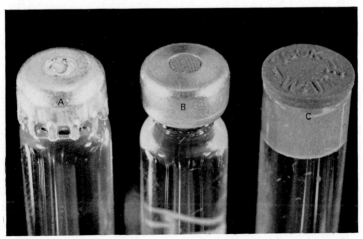

Fig. 16.—Different types of sealing cap for cartridges: **A**, Metal cap with soft metal centre; **B**, Metal cap with rubber centre; **C**, All-rubber sealing cap.

CARTRIDGES

Local anaesthetic solutions for use in dentistry are usually supplied pre-sterilized in cartridges and a typical example is illustrated in *Fig.* 9.

Alkali and pyrogen-free glass are used in the manufacture of these cartridges to avoid breakdown or contamination of the solution. The cartridges exhibit minor variations in design related mainly to the sealing cap which is pierced by the hypodermic needle when the syringe is loaded (*Fig.* 16).

Most cartridges contain either 2·2 ml. or 1·8 ml. of local anaesthetic solution. Cartridges of either size can be used in the standard syringe but 1·8 ml. of solution suffices for the average dental procedure. Since compression of the rubber plunger often produces slight aspiration when the pressure is released, contamination of the solution remaining in the cartridge can occur. For this reason residual solution must never be injected into a different patient because of the danger of cross-infection particularly that of hepatitis B associated antigen (HBsAg). Some wastage must, therefore, be accepted on many occasions when the larger cartridge is used.

NEEDLES

Hypodermic needles used in dentistry are usually classified as 'short' or 'long'. In the disposable range the short needles that are used for infiltration techniques are usually 2 cm. or 2·5 cm. in length whilst the needles employed for block techniques are usually 3·5 cm. long. The choice of needle should allow penetration to the depth required before its complete length has entered the tissues. This safety precaution leaves a length of needle protruding which, if fracture occurs at the hub, may be grasped with forceps or pliers and removed (*see* page 77).

The optimum gauge of the needles used for dental purposes is a matter of dispute. Many authorities believe that the use of a fine needle rather than a thicker one results in a more comfortable injection. Others suggest that fine needles are more liable to damage blood-vessels, muscles, and ligaments to produce haematomata and/or trismus (pages 73 and 74). It has also been claimed that certain tissues may deflect fine needles from a straight path of insertion and so predispose to the inaccurate placement of the solution. Nevertheless the authors, like most other dental surgeons, favour the use of fine needles of gauge 27. The even finer gauge 30 needles are excellent for use in infiltration techniques (page 37) but should not be used in inferior dental and other regional injections (page 45) because of the high risk of breakage within the tissues (page 77).

Whilst the acutely angled and double bevelled needle tip (*Fig.* 17) facilitates easy insertion into the tissues, it is easily damaged by contact with bone. This possibility provides a reason, in addition to the risk of cross-infection, why needles should be used on one occasion only.

STERILIZATION OF LOCAL ANAESTHETIC EQUIPMENT

Unless a dental surgeon possesses either an autoclave or hot-air sterilizer he can only disinfect metal syringes by using boiling water.

In the average dental surgery it is impossible to re-sterilize the lumen of a fine hypodermic needle prior to use without affecting the temper of the steel and increasing the risk of breakage. For this reason, the re-use of

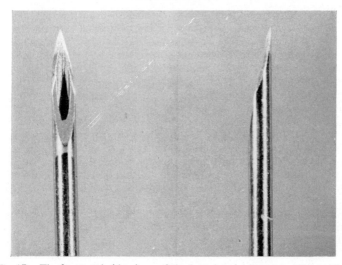

Fig. 17.—The front and side views of the long bevel with two additional bevels at the tip as used for most disposable needles.

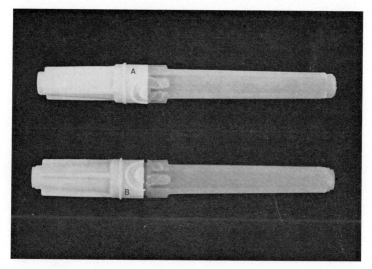

Fig. 18.—Plastic containers for disposable needles. **A**, Seal intact; **B**, Seal broken.

needles is to be deprecated for it is especially important to ensure that infection is not conveyed from one patient to another. In particular the risk of transmitting the virus which causes serum hepatitis places a grave responsibility upon the dental surgeon. These problems can be avoided by making it a rule never to use a hypodermic needle on more than one patient. The use of stainless-steel disposable needles is a most convenient way of attaining this objective. Such needles are pre-sterilized in plastic containers, the seals of which must be examined prior to use (*Fig.* 18). Needles in containers with a broken seal must be discarded.

Reputable manufacturers take stringent precautions to ensure that the local anaesthetic solutions that they supply are sterile. However, it is virtually certain that the outside of the cartridge will be contaminated by air-borne organisms or careless storage and handling. Sterilization of the 'needle' end of the cartridge must therefore be standard practice. Storage of cartridges in sterilizing solutions is contra-indicated because of the danger of contamination of the contents by seepage. Dry heat is the most effective means of sterilization which can be achieved by holding the sealed end of the cartridge in a gas jet for up to 5 seconds. This procedure has the added advantage of warming the solution and this may be continued by passing the cartridge back and forth through the flame four or five times. If discomfort during injection is to be avoided care must be taken to ensure that the solution is not over-heated.

Some manufacturers have introduced cartridges of solution that are sealed in individual compartments, in packs of five cartridges. Removal of a single cartridge and its immediate insertion into a sterile syringe virtually eliminates any risk of contamination of its surface.

CHAPTER VI

FUNDAMENTALS OF TECHNIQUE

THE importance of a quiet, confident, and friendly manner towards all patients cannot be over-emphasized. A smile and a few quiet words of welcome can pay dividends in the subsequent ease of management of the patient's treatment by establishing a base-line of trust.

Physical comfort is also essential for the co-operation of the patient and the ease of operation of the dental surgeon. *Fig.* 19 illustrates how the patient should be seated in a semi-reclining position with the back and legs supported and with the head-rest in the nape of the neck. The operator should stand on a non-slip surface, evenly balanced on both feet and as erect as is consistent with good vision of the injection site (*Fig.* 20). Those who operate with the patient in the supine position will need to modify their stance accordingly, but variations in the actual techniques of injection should be minimal.

PREMEDICATION

Most adult patients will respond to the dental surgeon's endeavours to gain his or her confidence and so premedication will not be required for the administration of a local anaesthetic for a relatively simple procedure.

However, some patients appreciate the support of drug therapy when coping with the stress of a visit to the dentist which their personality, imagination, or past experience has exaggerated. The nature and dosage of the premedicant drug and the route of administration will vary with the type of patient and the training and experience of the dentist.

Before premedication is undertaken careful inquiry must be made concerning any other medicines that the patient is receiving, for drugs may interact and potentiate the action of each other (page 80).

After the administration of any sedative drug he or she must not drive or ride any mechanically propelled machine or consume alcohol for the remainder of the working day.

The drugs suitable for administration by the oral route to dental patients may be chosen from a range which is conveniently subdivided as:— (1) *Non-barbiturate hypnotics;* (2) *Tranquillizers.*

Some tranquillizers may also be administered intravenously immediately prior to dental treatment.

Various preparations for oral administration which are included in the *Dental Practitioners' Formulary*, are listed in *Table III* (page 33) together with the adult doses. It must be emphasized that there is considerable individual variation in the reaction of patients to a given dosage of any drug. For this reason it is suggested that dental surgeons should become well acquainted with the use of a restricted number of drugs rather than have a superficial knowledge of a large variety of proprietary products.

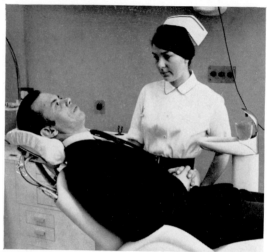

Fig. 19.—The patient in this photograph is comfortable. Note that the chair is tilted to a semi-reclining position, his back and shoulders are well supported, and the head-rest is in the nape of the neck.

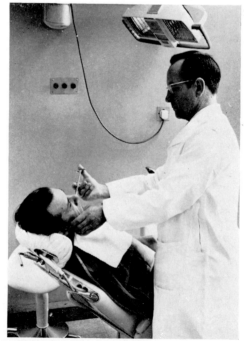

Fig. 20.—After the patient has been suitably draped the height of the chair is adjusted so that the operator has the light above and behind his right shoulder as he gives the injection.

The oral premedication of a really nervous patient should begin at least two and preferably three days before the dental appointment.

Although barbiturates have been used fairly extensively in the past it is now recognized that they may have severe limitations in producing tranquil sleep and actually lower the pain threshold. For these reasons they are not favoured by the authors for premedication of patients prior to the use of local anaesthesia.

However, preoperative apprehension may be controlled by the oral administration of a tranquillizer, for example, diazepam (Valium) 5–10 mg. before retiring on the three nights preceding the visit to the dentist and about 1 hour prior to the treatment.

Table III.—SEDATIVE DRUGS AVAILABLE FOR ORAL ADMINISTRATION WHICH ARE INCLUDED IN THE *Dental Practitioners' Formulary*

PROPRIETARY NAME	APPROVED NAME	AVERAGE ADULT DOSE
Non-barbiturates Welldorm Tricloryl	Dichloralphenazone Triclofos	1300 mg. (2 tablets) 1000 mg. (2 tablets)
Tranquillizers Librium Valium	Chlordiazepoxide Diazepam	} 5–10 mg. (1–2 tablets)
Equanil } Miltown }	Meprobamate	400 mg. (1 tablet)

Immediate sedation may be achieved in the dental surgery by the intravenous administration of a tranquillizing drug. Although a number of techniques are in existence, only that using diazepam will be described. This drug not only produces sedation but also slight muscular relaxation and some amnesia.

For intravenous injection diazepam is supplied in a 2-ml. ampoule of solution containing 10 mg. of the drug. The dose is 0·2 mg. per kg. of body-weight with a maximum of 20 mg. The injection should be made into a vein either at the lateral aspect of the ante-cubital fossa or in the back of the hand at the rate of 10 mg. in 60 seconds. The effect of that amount of the drug may then be assessed with the needle left in situ. A further quantity may then be injected if required. The assessment of adequate dosage is made from the patient's reactions of slight slurring of speech and a decreasing ability to focus the eyes. Drooping of the upper eyelids to a position half-way across the pupil (Verrill's sign, *Fig. 21*) is an indication that the maximum sedative dose has been administered. The sedative effect of the drug usually lasts about 45 minutes and during this time the patient should be co-operative and communicative. It is a wise precaution to keep the patient under surveillance for at least one hour after completion of the procedure because of postoperative drowsiness. He should also be warned that slight effects may last for the remainder of his working day so that he should not drive or ingest alcohol, anti-histamines, or sedatives during this period. Although there is minimal change in physiological processes under the influence of this drug it is wise, in the present state of knowledge, to confine its use in the dental chair to fit patients who have had nothing to eat or drink for 3–4 hours and who are escorted. The use of intra-venous diazepam in pregnant women should be avoided.

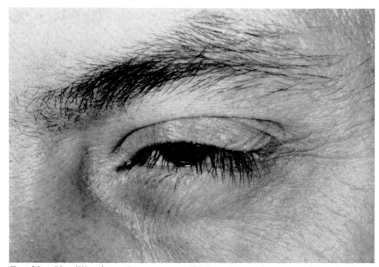

Fig. 21.—Verrill's sign: the upper eyelid has drooped to a position half-way across the pupil of the eye.

The local anaesthetic should be given immediately sedation is achieved because the amnesic effect of diazepam is greatest at this time. There is some evidence of depression of the laryngeal reflex, which is maximal during the first 5 minutes of sedation but has disappeared completely within 20 minutes. Therefore, adequate mouth packs must be used and suction apparatus utilized whenever this technique is employed (page 87).

Non-barbiturates or tranquillizers are particularly suitable for children because they are available in the form of elixirs (*see* page 37).

In practice it is found that many patients who require premedication at the first visit quickly overcome their apprehension and accept treatment without sedation at succeeding visits.

PREPARATION OF EQUIPMENT

As anticipation is often more disturbing than the actual treatment, few patients fail to appreciate the efficiency and speed with which a competent operator performs any dental procedure.

This is particularly true during the administration of a local anaesthetic when the ready availability and skilful use of equipment play a great part in impressing the patient with the ability of the operator. However, as many patients are upset by the mere sight of dental instruments care should be taken neither to flourish nor display them.

A typical lay-out of equipment and materials for the administration of a local anaesthetic is illustrated in *Fig.* 22.

Either a lighted gas jet or spirit lamp is used to flame the sealed end and warm the contents of a cartridge immediately prior to use. These objectives are obtained by rotating the cartridge through the flame several times as described on page 30.

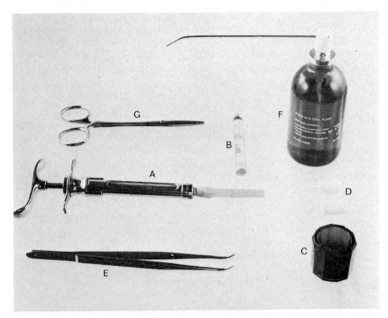

Fig. 22.—A typical lay-out of equipment and material required for the admini- stration of a local anaesthetic. A disposable syringe (A) ready for the insertion of the cartridge (B) after flaming. The Dappen glass (C) contains antiseptic solution for application on the cotton-wool rolls (D) held in the tweezers (E). Lignocaine anaesthetic spray (F) is ready if required. The Spencer Wells forceps (G) are readily accessible to remove a needle should it fracture at the hub.

The cartridge is then mounted in a previously sterilized syringe and the patency of the needle checked by expelling a small quantity of solution after removing the needle guard. The exact position of the bevel is adjusted so that it will face the bone on insertion and the guard replaced loosely. The assembled syringe is then put down in such a position that it can be picked up with one hand when required for use.

Whenever an injection is given, a pair of straight-nosed pliers or strong artery forceps should always be readily at hand (*Fig.* 22G) because on very rare occasions a needle may break at the hub. They are then available to grasp any part of a fractured needle that protrudes from the tissues (page 76).

Preparation of the Mucosa

As the mouth is constantly inhabited by a variety of micro-organisms, hypodermic injections through the oral mucosa may result in bacteria being introduced into the deeper tissues. The risk of infection from this source can be reduced by preparation of the mucosa in the following manner.

The area concerned is dried carefully with either gauze or cotton-wool and kept clear of further contamination with saliva by continued retraction of the soft tissues. Tincture of chlorhexidine 0·5 per cent on a cotton-wool roll is then applied to the site of injection for at least 15 seconds. Removal of surface epithelial cells by light 'scrubbing' of the area with the cotton-wool roll is not regarded as essential.

If surface anaesthesia is required it should be obtained in the manner described on page 38.

Speed of Injection

The ideal rate of injection varies with the density of the tissues at the site at which the solution is to be deposited and so it cannot be stated in precise terms. In general, the speed of injection is that which is consistent with the maximum comfort of the patient. Rapid injection of the solution may cause tissue distension and discomfort or actual cellular damage and pain when sensation returns. Furthermore, the risk of toxic reactions is greater if a quantity of anaesthetic agent is injected rapidly.

A slow rate of injection is thus essential and may be of the order of 1 ml. in 15 seconds when an infiltration technique is employed. For the inferior dental injection, however, 2 ml. may be injected in about 20 seconds after starting slowly, because the tissues in this area are of the loose areolar type in which distension is not the same problem as it is, for example, in the palate.

Testing for Anaesthesia

Altered sensation in itself is not a guarantee that anaesthesia has been achieved. When conservation procedures are undertaken the only certain method of testing that analgesia is complete is by cautious stimulation of the dentine with either a hand instrument or a bur.

Prior to the extraction of a tooth under local anaesthesia a dental probe may be pushed into the gingival crevice on both the labio-buccal and lingual surfaces of the root. The patient should be told that pressure may be felt and asked to state if 'sharpness' is noted. The presence of 'sharpness' is an indication for a further injection. The operator should not exhibit any doubt about the efficacy of his technique and avoid any mention of 'pain' if the confidence of his patient is not to be undermined.

The causes of failure to achieve anaesthesia are discussed on page 71.

Local Anaesthesia in Children

Few children look forward to visiting the dentist, especially when anaesthesia is to be used. Nevertheless, local anaesthesia is widely accepted by young dental patients, provided special attention is paid to certain points of technique. As the almost routine use of local anaesthesia can be a useful adjunct in gaining the co-operation of child patients, it should not be withheld until either pain or discomfort has been experienced. In the eyes of a child the white-coated dental surgeon often appears to be a large and forbidding figure. For this reason, he should arrange to be seated when he meets a child for the first time and attempt to initiate an appropriate non-dental conversation in the first instance. The child may then be told that it is necessary to put the tooth, and only the tooth, to sleep and be advised that the cheek or lips will feel 'rubbery' or 'tingly'. In many cases a rapport which facilitates treatment will readily be established whilst on other occasions the use of premedication will be indicated.

The sedation of a really nervous child should ensure a good sleep for two or three nights prior to the dental treatment. The drug of choice is diazepam elixir (Valium) in a dose of 2·5–5 mg. about half an hour before retiring to bed and a similar amount about one hour before the dental appointment. The intravenous form of diazepam may also be used immediately prior to treatment but the effects in children under 12 years of age are somewhat unpredictable. For this reason no dosages for the intravenous route are included in this text and special training in the technique is recommended.

Sedation may also be achieved by using a hypnotic such as chloral elixir paediatric B.P.C., which contains 200 mg. chloral hydrate in 5 ml. The dose recommended for a child aged between 1 and 5 years is 5–7·5 ml. (1–1½ British Standard spoonfuls). An alternative preparation is triclofos elixir B.P.C. (Tricloryl Syrup), which contains 500 mg. triclofos sodium in 5 ml., and which is given to children aged 1–5 years in a dosage of 2·5–5 ml. (½–1 British Standard spoonful).

The regimen of administration should be similar to that recommended for diazepam elixir but with only half of the individual dose given 1 hour before the dental visit.

The use of surface anaesthesia, unless contra-indicated, and of infiltration techniques employing 30 gauge needles and warm solution should reduce discomfort to a minimum. If the child is frightened by the sensation of local anaesthesia it usually helps if a hand mirror is used to demonstrate that the face is normal, despite the affected area feeling swollen. Continuous verbal encouragement should be given in the course of treatment by the dental surgeon, but care should be taken to avoid the use of emotive words such as 'hurt', 'needle', 'prick', even in the negative sense, e.g. 'This won't hurt'! Gentle physical contact with the dental surgery assistant. e.g., holding hands, often enhances the co-operation of the child as do complimentary remarks concerning his behaviour during and after treatment. It should never be necessary to force local anaesthesia on a child who objects to its use, as sedation or even general anaesthesia provide acceptable alternatives.

TYPES OF LOCAL ANAESTHESIA

For descriptive purposes it is convenient to sub-divide local anaesthesia on an anatomical basis into topical, infiltration, and regional techniques (page 9).

1. Topical or Surface Anaesthesia.—Topical anaesthesia is obtained by the application of a suitable anaesthetic agent to an area of either skin or mucous membrane which it penetrates to anaesthetize superficial nerve-endings (*see Fig.* 3A, p. 10). It is most commonly used to obtain anaesthesia of mucosa prior to injection. *Sprays* containing an appropriate local anaesthetic agent (*see* page 18) are particularly suitable for this purpose because of their rapidity of action. The active ingredient is 10 per cent lignocaine hydrochloride in a water miscible base, which is expelled in small quantities from an aerosol container (*see Fig.* 22F, p. 35). The inclusion of various fruit flavours is intended to make such preparations more acceptable to children but may present problems due to the excessive salivation which they may stimulate.

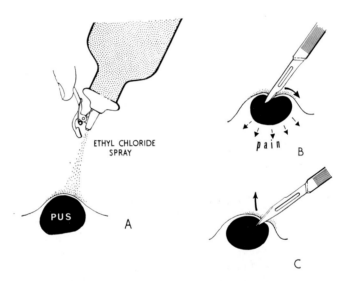

Fig. 23.—A, When used to produce refrigeration anaesthesia, ethyl chloride spray anaesthetizes only the overlying tissues which are covered with 'snow'. B, Downwards pressure with a No. 15 blade causes pain by increasing pressure within the abscess. C, Pain can be avoided by using a No. 11 blade with an outwards motion. (*From* '*Minor Oral Surgery*', 2nd ed., by Geoffrey L. Howe, Bristol, Wright, 1971.)

When used as a spray it is very easy to spread the solution, and its effect, much more extensively than is desired. It is preferable, after drying the area concerned, to spray an appropriate quantity of solution on to a small cotton-wool roll which is placed at the injection site in the sulcus and left in situ for about a minute prior to insertion of the needle. Preparation of the mucosa is not required since anaesthetic sprays have an antiseptic effect. The onset time of anaesthesia is approximately 1 minute and the duration round about 10 minutes.

Ointments containing 5 per cent lignocaine hydrochloride can be used for a similar purpose but take 3–4 minutes to produce surface anaesthesia.

Some manufacturers include in their products an enzyme, hyaluronidase, which is said to aid penetration of the tissues by the local anaesthetic agent. Amethocaine and benzocaine are included in other preparations. Ointments are particularly useful when applied to tender gingivae prior to deep scaling.

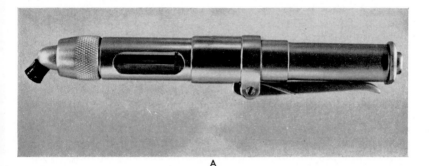

A

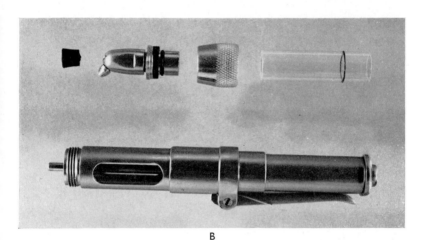

B

Fig. 24.—A, A 'Panjet' instrument assembled for use. B, The dismantled instrument showing (left to right) rubber cone, nozzle, nozzle-retaining ring, and glass reservoir. Below this is the casing with cocking handle underneath and the trigger stud at the end on the right.

An *emulsion* containing 2 per cent lignocaine hydrochloride is also available. This is of value when full-mouth impressions have to be taken in patients who are prone to retching. One teaspoonful should be washed round the mouth and oro-pharynx for a minute or two and any excess spat out immediately prior to the impression being taken. It is also useful for the relief of postoperative tenderness such as that following a gingivectomy and is quite safe if swallowed inadvertently.

Ethyl chloride when sprayed on to either skin or mucosa volatilizes so rapidly that it quickly produces anaesthesia by refrigeration. This phenomenon is of clinical value only when the spray is directed at a limited area until 'snow' appears. Care must be taken to avoid stimulation of the pulps of adjacent teeth and undue inhalation of the vapour by the patient. This technique is of limited value but is occasionally used to produce surface anaesthesia prior to the incision of fluctuant abscesses (*Fig.* 23).

'*Jet injection*' is a technique in which a small amount of local anaesthetic solution is propelled as a jet into the sub-mucosa without the use of a hypodermic needle.

Most of the instruments used for this purpose, including the example illustrated in *Fig.* 24, have to be 'primed' and 'cocked' prior to use and depend upon the discharge of a small quantity of local anaesthetic solution from a reservoir. This takes place when a knob is pressed to release air pressure which produces a very fine jet of solution which penetrates the mucosa through a small puncture wound to produce surface anaesthesia. The hypodermic needle is then inserted painlessly through the same wound. This technique is particularly effective prior to palatal injections since other methods produce only partial anaesthesia in this site, but some patients object to the popping sound when the instrument is fired.

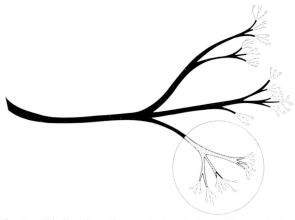

Fig. 25.—Local infiltration of anaesthetic solution will anaesthetize the nerve-fibres in a small area (represented by the light shading within the circle) but leave the remainder of the nerve unaffected.

2. Infiltration Anaesthesia.—Anaesthetic solution deposited near the terminal fibres of any nerve will infiltrate through the tissues to reach the nerve-fibres and thus produce anaesthesia of the localized area served by them (*Fig.* 25). This infiltration technique is further sub-divided into:—

a. Sub-mucous Injection.—This term is applied when the solution is deposited just beneath the mucous membrane. Whilst this is unlikely to produce anaesthesia of the dental pulp it is often employed either to anaesthetize the long buccal nerve prior to the extraction of mandibular molars (*see Fig.* 58, p. 64) or for soft tissue surgery.

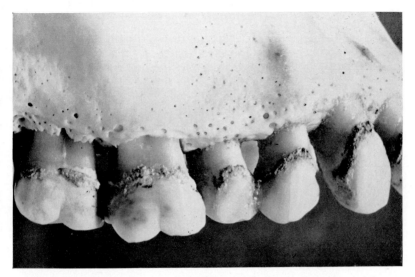

A

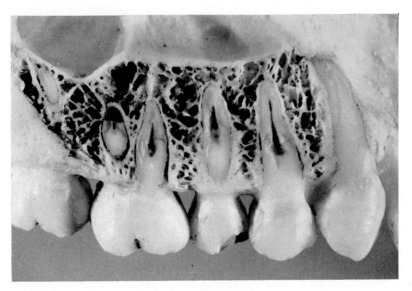

B

Fig. 26.—Alveolar bone of the maxilla. A, Perforation of the cortical plate by vascular canals is apparent. B, Some of the outer cortical plate has been removed to demonstrate its thinness. (Compare with *Fig.* 32, p. 45.)

b. Supra-periosteal Injection.—In some sites, such as the maxilla, the outer cortical plate of alveolar bone is thin and perforated by tiny vascular canals (*Fig.* 26). In these areas when anaesthetic solution is deposited outside the periosteum it will infiltrate through the periosteum, cortical plate, and medullary bone to the nerve-fibres. By this means anaesthesia of the dental pulp can be obtained by injecting alongside the approximate position of the tooth apex (*Fig.* 27). The supra-periosteal injection is the technique most frequently used in dentistry and is often loosely described as 'infiltration'.

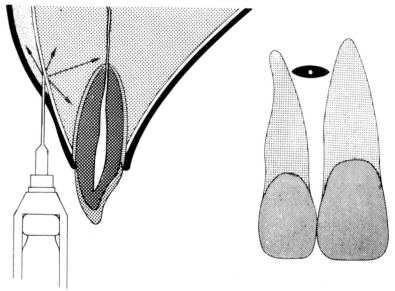

Fig. 27.—When making a supra-periosteal injection the local anaesthetic solution is deposited outside the periosteum. It will then infiltrate through the periosteum and alveolar bone, as indicated by the arrows, to reach the nerve-fibres supplying the tooth and supporting tissues.

Fig. 28.—Intra-osseous technique. Incision of the muco-periosteum and perforation of the outer cortical plate with a bur hole in a position between the roots of the teeth to be anaesthetized.

c. Sub-periosteal Injection.—In this technique the anaesthetic solution is deposited between the periosteum and the cortical plate. As these structures are firmly bound together this injection is painful. Therefore it should only be used if there is no alternative or when superficial anaesthesia has been achieved by a supra-periosteal injection. This technique can be of value if a supra-periosteal injection has failed to produce complete anaesthesia.

d. Intra-osseous Injection.—As the name implies, in this technique the solution is deposited within the medullary bone. The procedure is most effectively carried out by the use of bone drills and needles especially designed for the purpose. After giving a supra-periosteal injection in the ordinary way a very small incision is made through the muco-periosteum at the chosen site of injection to provide access for the introduction of a bur or fine reamer. A small hole is then made through the outer cortical plate of bone with the instrument selected. The siting of this hole is critical and is illustrated in *Fig.* 28. It must be near the apex of the tooth concerned but in such a position that damage cannot be caused to the roots of the teeth.

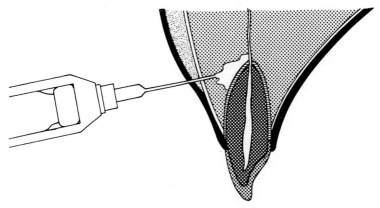

Fig. 29.—The needle is inserted through the bur hole and the local anaesthetic solution injected into the medullary bone through which it infiltrates readily.

A short needle supported by a long hub is inserted through the hole and advanced into the bone. 0·25 ml of anaesthetic solution is then deposited slowly in the medullary spaces of the bone (*Fig.* 29). This amount of solution is usually sufficient for most dental procedures. The intraosseous technique produces excellent anaesthesia of the pulp accompanied by minimal impairment of sensation in the soft tissues. However, some trauma to the alveolar bone is inevitable and a potential route for infection is produced. Strict attention to asepsis at all stages of the procedure is mandatory. In practice the effectiveness of the anaesthetic solutions now available has reduced considerably the need for intra-osseus injections and the technique is seldom used.

e. Intra-septal Injection.—This modified version of the intra-osseous technique is sometimes used when difficulty in gaining complete anaesthesia is experienced, or when an immediate denture is to be fitted and supra-periosteal techniques are best avoided. A gauge 27 needle is thrust into the soft bone at the alveolar crest (*Fig.* 30). The solution is injected under pressure and passes through the medullary bone and periodontal tissues to produce anaesthesia. This technique should only be used after superficial anaesthesia has been obtained. In view of the needle trauma and the possibility of infection spreading from the gingivae it should not be used to produce local anaesthesia for cavity preparation.

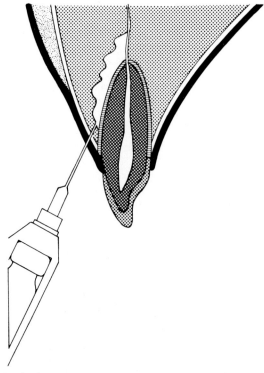

Fig. 30.—In the intra-septal technique the needle is thrust into the medullary bone near the alveolar crest. Local anaesthetic solution injected in this position infiltrates readily towards the apex of the tooth.

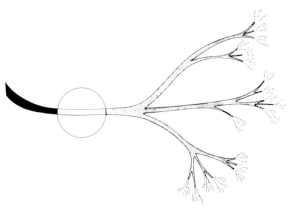

Fig. 31.—If local anaesthetic solution is injected near a nerve trunk, e.g., within the circle, all impulses from the distribution of that nerve will be 'blocked' and regional anaesthesia achieved.

3. Regional Anaesthesia.—Anaesthetic solution deposited near a nerve trunk will, by blocking all impulses, produce anaesthesia of the area supplied by that nerve. This is known as 'regional' or 'block' anaesthesia (*Fig.* 31).

Although this technique may be used in the maxilla it is of particular

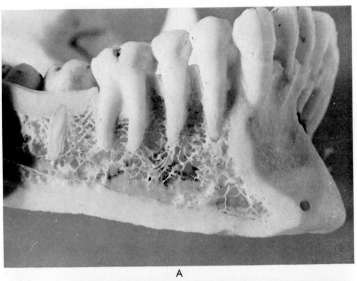

A

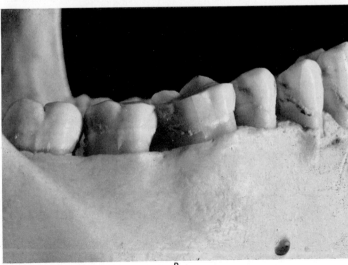

B

Fig. 32.—Mandibular alveolar bone. The outer cortical plate is thick (A) and devoid of vascular canals (B). It is therefore comparatively impervious to infiltration of anaesthetic solutions. (Compare with *Fig.* 26, page 41.)

value in dentistry for producing anaesthesia in the mandible. The use of infiltration technique in the mandible is unreliable due to the density of the outer cortical plate of bone (*Fig.* 32). By placing the anaesthetic solution in the pterygo-mandibular space near the mandibular foramen (*Fig.* 50, page 59) regional anaesthesia over the whole distribution of the inferior dental nerve on that side is obtained.

CHAPTER VII

LOCAL ANAESTHESIA IN THE MAXILLA

THE oral cavity is one of the most sensitive parts of the body. Sensory nerve-endings are present in the dental pulp, the periodontal ligament, the alveolar bone, the muco-periosteum, and the mucous membrane.

In the maxilla it is convenient to regard the innervation as consisting of an outer nerve loop and an inner nerve loop. The former is composed of nerve fibrils which originate in the teeth and their labio-buccal supporting tissues and form a plexus in the bone above the apices.

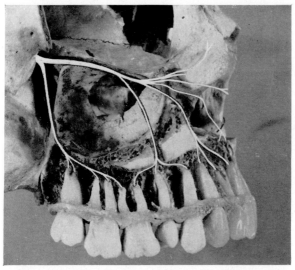

Fig. 33.—Outer nerve loop. The area of distribution of the maxillary nerve. The lateral wall of the maxillary sinus has been removed.

From this plexus, superior dental nerves ascend in bony canals to join the infra-orbital or maxillary nerves, the central connexions of which have been described already (page 3). Despite the presence of this anastomosis it is generally accepted that for all practical purposes the innervation of the teeth in the anterior, middle, and posterior parts of the maxilla is as shown in *Fig.* 33 and detailed below.

Analgesia of the outer nerve loop suffices for cavity preparation in most cases, but surgical procedures involving the palatal supporting tissues necessitate anaesthesia of the inner nerve loop (page 53) in addition.

ANAESTHESIA OF THE PERMANENT CHEEK TEETH

The upper third molar, second molar, and the disto-buccal and palatal roots of the first molar are innervated by branches which form the posterior superior dental nerve (*Fig.* 34). Small branches of the same nerve transmit sensation from the buccal supporting tissues in the molar region and the

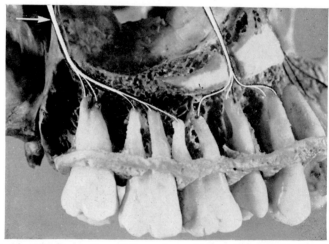

Fig. 34.—The innervation of the molar and premolar teeth via the posterior superior dental nerve and the middle superior dental nerve. The arrow indicates the position of the foramen through which the former leaves the upper part of the tuberosity.

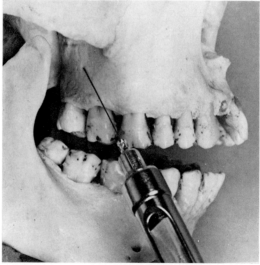

Fig. 35.—The position of the needle for infiltration of the porous area of bone between the second and third molars.

muco-periosteum attached to them. Deposition of anaesthetic solution close to the nerve after it leaves its bony canal produces regional anaesthesia of the structures it supplies. This technique is known as *the posterior superior dental block*. Since the introduction of modern local anaesthetic agents it is more usual to employ infiltration techniques in this area because the deposition of about 1 ml. of solution in the position illustrated in *Fig.* 35 normally produces adequate anaesthesia without the risk of damage to the pterygoid venous plexus (page 73).

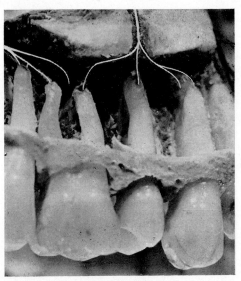

Fig. 36.—Nerve-fibres from the disto-buccal and palatal roots of the upper first molar ascend in the posterior superior dental nerve. Those from the mesio-buccal root join the middle superior dental nerve.

The mesio-buccal root of the first molar, both premolars, and the buccal supporting tissues and muco-periosteum related to them are innervated via the middle superior dental nerve (*Fig.* 36). Infiltration techniques are usually employed to anaesthetize these structures. Deposition of 1 ml. of solution in the position shown in *Figs.* 37 and 38 suffices to anaesthetize the outer nerve loop supplying the second premolar.

A similar technique should suffice to anaesthetize the first premolar but may not be adequate for the first molar. This is because the buccal bone of the zygomatic process is dense and is perforated by comparatively few vascular canals (*Fig.* 37). The density of this bone may impede the penetration of the outer plate by the local anaesthetic solution and so it is often necessary to give two injections in the more porous sites illustrated in *Figs.* 35 and 37 in order to obtain effective anaesthesia of the first molar.

ANAESTHESIA OF THE PERMANENT ANTERIOR TEETH

The upper incisor and canine teeth are innervated by fibres which form the anterior superior dental nerve (*Fig.* 39). This nerve ascends in a fine bony canal to join the infra-orbital nerve about 0·5 cm. inside the infra-orbital canal. The central incisor, lateral incisor, or canine may be anaes-thetized, together with their supporting tissues, by depositing about 1 ml. of local anaesthetic solution near the apex of the tooth concerned. *Fig.* 40 shows the correct site of the needle when the upper lateral incisor is being anaesthetized. The ease with which the floor of the nose may be penetrated due to miscalculation of the length of the root or the depth of the labial sulcus is shown in *Fig.* 41.

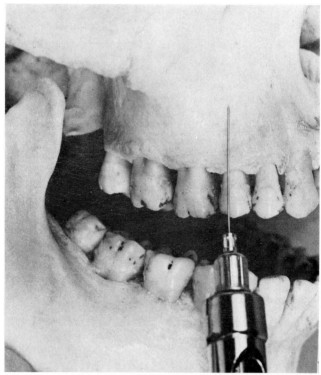

Fig. 37.—The position of the needle for infiltration of the upper second premolar.

ANAESTHESIA OF THE PALATAL TISSUES

Nerve-endings in the palatal soft tissues related to the anterior maxillary teeth and premaxilla transmit sensation via nerve-fibrils which unite to form the long spheno-palatine nerve. This passes through the incisive foramen and canal and then upwards and backwards across the nasal septum to reach the spheno-palatine ganglion (*Figs.* 42, 43).

Numerous small branches from the palatal gingivae and muco-periosteum in the premolar and molar regions unite to form the greater palatine nerve. After passing backwards in a bony channel situated approximately

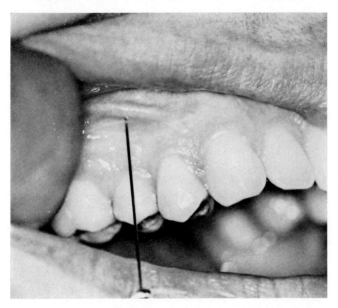

Fig. 38.—To achieve anaesthesia of the upper second premolar the injection is made just above the upper limit of the attached mucosa with the needle in line with the long axis of the tooth.

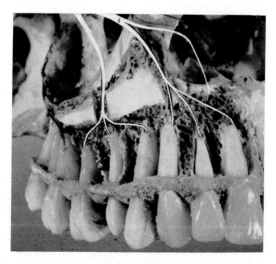

Fig. 39.—The path of the anterior superior dental nerve from the upper canine and incisor teeth.

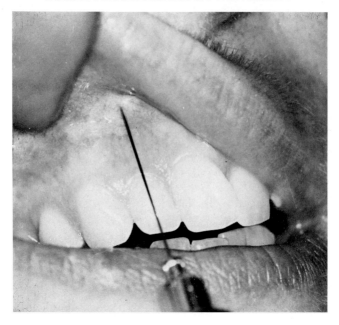

Fig. 40.—An infiltration injection in line with the long axis of the upper lateral incisor illustrates the point of insertion of the needle and the importance of pulling the lip outwards to make the tissues taut. They may then be drawn downwards on to the point of the needle as it is pushed firmly upwards.

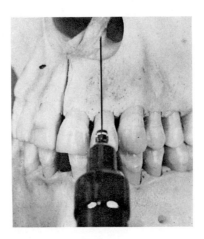

Fig. 41.—The floor of the nose is reached easily if the tip of a long disposable needle is inserted too deeply.

half-way between the midline of the palate and the gingival margin of the teeth, this nerve enters its canal through the greater palatine foramen (*Fig.* 42). It then ascends to join the spheno-palatine ganglion which is connected to the maxillary nerve (*Fig.* 44).

The long spheno-palatine and greater palatine nerves anastomose in the canine region of the palate and constitute the inner nerve loop.

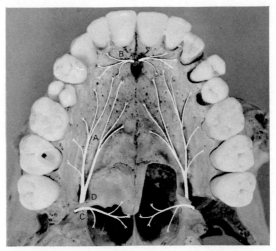

Fig. 42.—The complete innervation of the palate showing the anastomosis of the greater palatine (**A**) and long spheno-palatine nerves (**B**) in the region of the first premolar. Note the close proximity of the lesser palatine nerve (**C**) to the greater palatine foramen (**D**)

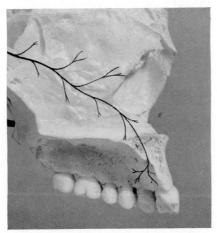

Fig. 43.—The approximate path of the long spheno-palatine nerve ascending across the nasal septum from the premaxilla.

The palatal muco-periosteum is firm in consistency and is closely adapted to the bone. These characteristics make it necessary to inject local anaesthetic solutions under greater pressure than is required in other sites. For this reason patients should be warned prior to injection that palatal injections cause some discomfort if not actual pain. This may be minimized by inserting the needle with the bevel facing the bone and as near as possible at right angles to the vault of the palate as illustrated in *Fig.* 45. In the premaxilla, injection into the incisive papilla is extremely painful and should be avoided (*Fig.* 46).

Palatal injections are usually given over the estimated position of the apex of the tooth to be anaesthetized. However, care should be taken to avoid injecting solution too close to the greater palatine foramen as the lesser palatine nerve may be affected (*Fig.* 42). This will produce anaesthesia of the soft palate, tonsillar and uvular areas making swallowing difficult and causing unnecessary discomfort or distress to the patient. For this reason palatal injections should never be given posterior to the second molar tooth. Injections directly into palatal foramina should also be

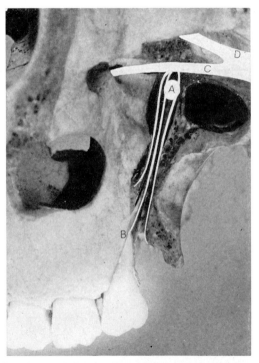

Fig. 44.—The spheno-palatine ganglion (A) showing the greater palatine nerve (B) joining it from the greater palatine canal between the posterior-superior dental nerve anteriorly and lesser palatine nerve posteriorly. Branches from the ganglion join the maxillary nerve (C) to connect with the trigeminal ganglion (D).

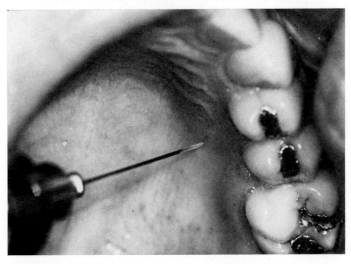

Fig. 45.—Palatal injection in the premolar area. Note the insertion of the needle from the opposite side of the mouth at right angles to the vault of the palate and about half-way between the midline of the palate and the gingival margin.

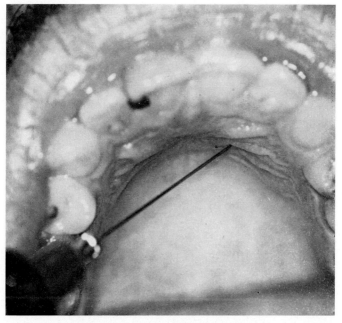

Fig. 46.—Palatal injection in the premaxilla. Infiltration of a site lateral to the central rugae and slow deposition of the anaesthetic solution aid significantly the comfort of the patient.

avoided due to the risk of damage to the nerve (page 74) or intra-vascular injection (page 73).

ANAESTHESIA OF THE DECIDUOUS TEETH

In children, multiple vascular canals perforate the thin labio-buccal alveolar plate. For this reason infiltration techniques are highly effective in producing anaesthesia of upper deciduous teeth. Care should be taken to avoid the mistake of misjudging the length of the roots and inserting the needle too deeply into the tissues.

In young children the discomfort of a palatal injection for the extraction of a tooth or the placement of a matrix band may be avoided in the following manner:—

After a supra-periosteal injection in the labio-buccal sulcus has taken effect, injections are made from the labio-buccal aspect, via the related interproximal spaces, at the level at which the gingival tissues are attached to the underlying periosteum. The small amounts of solution deposited in this way will provide adequate anaesthesia of the palatal tissues.

THE INFRA-ORBITAL INJECTION

Since infiltration techniques are so effective in the maxilla, regional anaesthesia is seldom required. However, the infra-orbital injection may be of value if numerous extractions or extensive surgery are to be undertaken in the maxillary incisor and canine regions. It may also be employed for anaesthetizing an anterior tooth where the use of infiltration technique is precluded by the presence of infection at the site of injection.

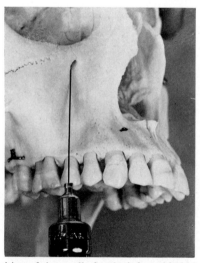

Fig. 47.—The position of the needle for the infra-orbital block by the intra-oral route. Note that the syringe is in the long axis of the second upper premolar.

This technique is based upon the fact that solution deposited at the orifice of the infra-orbital foramen (*Fig.* 47) passes along the canal to involve both the anterior and middle superior dental nerves thus producing anaesthesia of the incisor, canine, and premolar teeth and their supporting structures. While the solution sometimes reaches the spheno-palatine ganglion and anaesthetizes the inner nerve loop, supplementary palatal injections are often required.

Either an intra-oral or an extra-oral approach may be employed for the infra-orbital block. The intra-oral technique is more popular and allows the needle to be kept out of the patient's sight. It is performed in the following manner.

The infra-orbital ridge is palpated and the infra-orbital notch located with the tip of the first finger, which is then moved slightly downwards to lie directly over the infra-orbital foramen. With the finger-tip maintained in that position the thumb is used to reflect the upper lip and expose the site of injection (*Fig.* 48).

After preparing the mucosa (page 36) the tip of a long needle is inserted just above the reflection of the mucous membrane over the apex of the

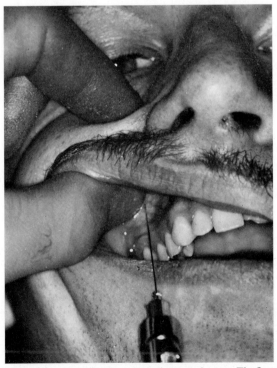

Fig. 48.—The infra-orbital injection via the intra-oral route. The first finger of the left hand is palpating the foramen whilst the thumb is retracting the buccal tissues and the needle is advanced close to bone in line with the long axis of the second upper premolar.

second premolar. The needle is advanced in line with the long axis of this tooth to a depth of 1·5–2 cm. The correct position of the tip of the needle overlying the foramen is confirmed when the injection of solution is felt beneath the palpating fingertip (*Fig.* 48). The deposition of 1 ml. suffices in most instances.

Throughout this procedure the needle must be kept in close proximity to the outer surface of the periosteum in order to minimize the risk of piercing the infra-orbital plexus of veins and so producing a haematoma (page 73).

When the extra-oral method is employed the infra-orbital foramen is located in the manner previously described, the patient told to close his eyes, and the overlying skin prepared by 'scrubbing' for at least 15 seconds with tincture of chlorhexidine 0·5 per cent on a gauze swab. The tip of a short needle is then inserted at the angle illustrated in *Fig.* 49 until it lies at the foramen, care being taken to ensure that it does not enter the canal. 1 ml. of solution is then deposited. Although anaesthesia of the soft tissues will be immediate, at least 2 minutes should elapse before testing for anaesthesia of the dental structures (page 36).

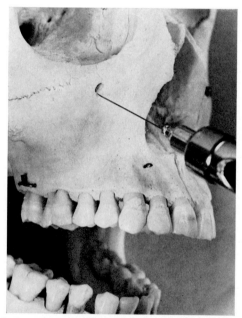

Fig. 49.—Angulation of the needle for the extra-oral approach to the infra-orbital block injection to avoid entry into the infra-orbital canal.

CHAPTER VIII

LOCAL ANAESTHESIA IN THE MANDIBLE

As in the maxilla it is convenient to regard the innervation of the mandible as consisting of outer and inner nerve loops. The former is composed of nerve fibrils which originate in the teeth and their labio-buccal supporting tissues. These fibrils combine to form the inferior dental and long buccal nerves.

The inner nerve loop is composed of nerve-fibrils which arise in the lingual muco-periosteum and mucosa and combine with fibrils from the anterior two-thirds of the tongue to form the lingual nerve.

All these nerves pass backwards and upwards to join the mandibular division of the trigeminal nerve, the central connexions of which have been described on page 3. Analgesia of the inferior dental nerve alone suffices for cavity preparation in most cases but surgical procedures involve the supporting tissues and require anaesthesia of both the inner and outer nerve loops.

THE PTERYGO-MANDIBULAR SPACE

Due to the density of the buccal plate bone infiltration techniques are of limited value in the mandible and regional or block anaesthesia is most frequently employed. This is achieved by the deposition of solution around the inferior dental and lingual nerves in the pterygo-mandibular space (*Fig.* 50). A detailed knowledge of the anatomy of this area is essential (*Figs.* 51 and 52).

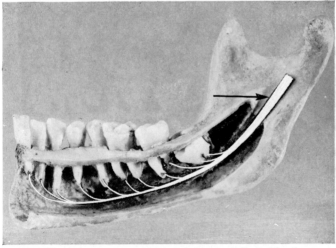

Fig. 50.—Injection of local anaesthetic solution, as indicated by the arrow, near the mandibular foramen will produce regional anaesthesia of the inferior dental nerve on that side.

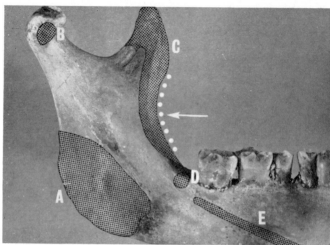

Fig. 51.—Attachments to the medial aspect of the mandible of significance in local anaesthetic techniques. **A,** Medial pterygoid muscle; **B,** Lateral pterygoid muscle; **C,** Temporalis muscle; **D,** Pterygo-mandibular raphe; **E,** Mylo-hyoid muscle. The dotted line indicates the coronoid notch and the arrow its deepest point.

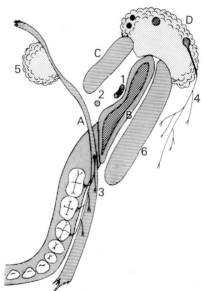

Fig. 52.—The pterygo-mandibular space is bounded by: **A,** Posterior fibres of buccinator muscles and anterior fibres of superior constrictor muscle which are both attached to the pterygo-mandibular raphe; **B,** The ascending ramus of the mandible; **C,** The medial pterygoid muscle; **D,** The parotid gland.

The nerves associated with it are: **1,** The inferior dental nerve; **2,** The lingual nerve; **3,** The long buccal nerve. Other structures shown are: **4,** The facial nerve; **5,** The tonsil; **6,** The masseter muscle.

The space is bounded anteriorly by the pterygo-mandibular raphe and the fibres of superior constrictor and buccinator muscles that are inserted into it. The posterior boundary is formed by the parotid gland. The inner surface of the ascending ramus of the mandible forms the lateral wall whilst the medial pterygoid muscle forms its floor and deep boundary. The lateral pterygoid muscle constitutes the 'roof' of the space (*Fig.* 51). The lingual nerve ascends diagonally backwards and upwards through the space, passing just in front of the inferior dental nerve (*Fig.* 52) as the latter emerges from the mandibular foramen (*Fig.* 51). A shallow bony depression just above the foramen is the site in which solution should be deposited for an inferior dental block.

The long buccal nerve is composed of fibrils arising in the cheek and buccal muco-periosteum in the molar region. After crossing the anterior border of the ascending ramus it traverses the upper part of the space to join the anterior division of the mandibular nerve. It is thus remote from the mandibular foramen and a separate injection is necessary when anaesthesia of the buccal soft tissue in the molar region is required (page 63).

The Inferior Dental Injection

By blocking the inferior dental and lingual nerves on one side, together with the long buccal nerve where necessary, it is possible to obtain anaesthesia from the third molar to the canine. The success of this technique is

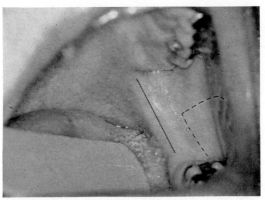

Fig. 53.—The surface markings of the buccal pad of fat (broken) and the mucosa covering the pterygo-mandibular raphe (continuous).

almost entirely dependent upon the accurate deposition of solution. This may be accomplished in the following manner.

The patient is seated in the chair and the head-rest adjusted so that his mandibular occlusal plane is almost horizontal when the mouth is open (*Fig.* 19, page 32). The dentist should stand in front of his patient for the right inferior dental block and behind the chair whilst giving an injection on the opposite side. Upon intra-oral inspection it is usually possible to identify the distal angle or apex of the buccal pad of fat and also the ridge of mucous membrane covering the pterygo-mandibular raphe (*Fig.* 53).

As this latter structure passes upwards and inwards from the posterior end of the mylo-hyoid line of the mandible to the hamulus of the medial ptery-goid plate, the point of insertion should always be lateral to and in front of it. The point of insertion will usually coincide with the apex of the buccal pad but since the position of this structure is variable it is necessary to confirm the visual landmarks by palpation.

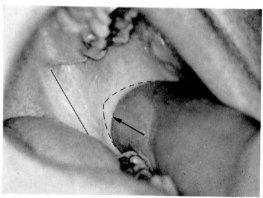

Fig. 54.—The palpating thumb (or finger) in the retro-molar depression coincides at the mid-point of the nail with the apex of the buccal pad.

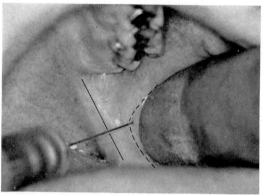

Fig 55.—Insertion of the needle from a position approximately over the lower premolars of the opposite side and just beyond the mid-point of the nail.

The thumb of the left hand is passed along the buccal surfaces of the lower molar teeth until the external oblique ridge is felt. The tip is then 'rolled' inwards to lie in the retro-molar fossa (*Fig.* 54).

The mid-point of the nail should then lie in the deepest part of the coronoid notch at the level of the mandibular fossa (*Fig.* 51). This position usually coincides with the apex of the buccal pad of fat and the internal oblique line. After preparation of the mucosa a long needle is inserted at this point (*Fig.* 55).

With the barrel of the syringe held parallel to the mandibular occlusal plane and over the second premolar tooth of the opposite side of the mouth the tip of the needle is inserted for about 0·5 cm and a few drops of solution are injected there to anaesthetize the lingual nerve (*Fig.* 56). This step may be omitted when analgesia is required for conservative procedures unless extensive preparations are being undertaken which involve the lingual gingivae.

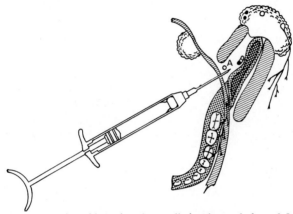

Fig. 56.—From the point of insertion the needle is advanced about 0·5 cm. and a few drops injected to anaesthetize the lingual nerve (A).

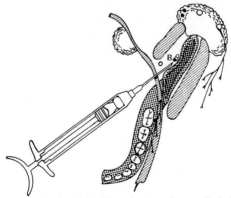

Fig. 57.—After anaesthesia of the lingual nerve the needle is inserted a further 1·5–2 cm. and should then be very near the inferior dental bundle (B) before the latter enters the mandibular foramen.

The needle should be advanced gently for a further 1·5–2 cm. until its tip lightly contacts the bone above the mandibular foramen (*Fig.* 57). It is then withdrawn slightly and about 1·5 ml. of solution deposited (*Fig.* 57). The syringe is then withdrawn steadily keeping the needle straight.

The solution remaining in the cartridge is used to produce infiltration anaesthesia of the long buccal nerve if it is required. This may be achieved by means of a sub-mucous injection in which the solution is deposited either in the buccal sulcus just posterior to the molar tooth involved (*Fig.* 58) or high in the retro-molar fossa. Such injections will anaesthetize not only the gingivae but also the inner aspect of the cheek as far forwards as the corner of the mouth.

The technique described for anaesthetizing the inferior dental nerve is known as 'the direct method' in contra-distinction to 'the indirect method' in earlier texts. Since the introduction of thinner needles the latter more complex approach is seldom used because of the danger of bending the fine, flexible needles within the tissues.

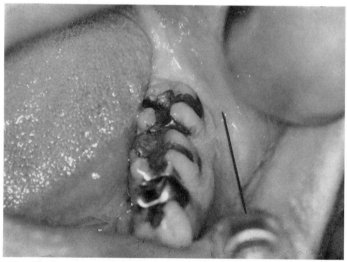

Fig. 58.—The long buccal injection is made just posterior and buccal to the last molar tooth which is about to be extracted.

The speed of onset of anaesthesia is variable but will be heralded by a change of sensation in the tongue and lower lip when compared with the opposite side. This symptom may be described by different patients as 'pins and needles', 'frozen', 'wooden', 'swollen', etc. It is often necessary to wait for three or four minutes after these initial changes before surgical anaesthesia can be guaranteed.

On rare occasions there may be a clinical indication for the use of bilateral inferior dental injections. However, it is the opinion of the authors that bilateral mandibular anaesthesia should be employed only by very experienced operators treating carefully selected patients.

Whilst many patients will accept bilateral local anaesthesia in the maxilla, the wide distribution of soft tissue anaesthesia following an inferior dental injection warrants careful consideration before bilateral mandibular anaesthesia is undertaken. If clinical considerations demand bilateral injections, the psychological make-up of the patient must be a prime factor in the management of the problem since complete loss of sensation in the tongue has been known to provoke a disturbing hysterical response. Furthermore, the risk of self-inflicted soft tissue damage by the patient must be enhanced. For these reasons bilateral inferior dental injections should be avoided whenever possible.

The dimensions and shape of the mandible may vary in patients of differing race, size, and age. Thus the width of the ascending ramus and hence the position of the mandibular foramen may vary between different individuals. For this reason it is often helpful to palpate both the anterior and posterior borders of the ascending ramus as shown in *Fig.* 59. The

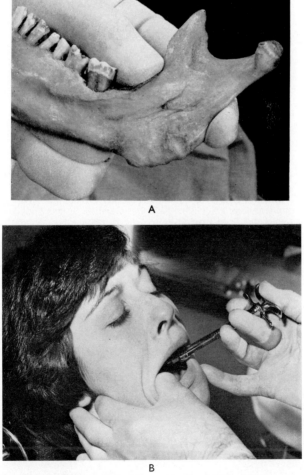

A

B

Fig. 59.—If the thumb is used for intra-oral palpation the first (or second) finger may be used to palpate the angle and posterior border of the ascending ramus as an aid to determining its width. A, On a mandible; B, On a patient.

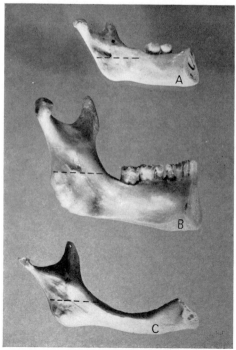

Fig. 60.—Mesial aspect of the mandible of a 6-year-old child (A), average adult (B), and an edentulous adult (C). Note the variation in size and shape of the ascending ramus and the relative position of the mandibular foramen to the occlusal plane.

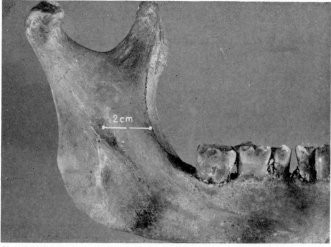

Fig. 61.—Mesial aspect of the ascending ramus of an average adult showing the distance between the internal oblique ridge and the inferior dental foramen.

needle may then be inserted as previously described and directed midway between the finger and thumb.

A similar approach may be employed if it is necessary to give an inferior dental block to a very young child. A short needle should be used in such a case and inserted in a slightly downward direction, so that the tip of the needle is more closely related to the mandibular foramen (*Fig.* 60A).

In the elderly edentulous patient gross resorption may alter the relative relationship of the mandibular foramen. As a general rule the point of insertion of the needle will be somewhat higher than in the dentate patient and is best determined by palpating the coronoid notch (*Fig.* 60C).

The distance from the internal oblique line to the mandibular foramen seldom exceeds 2 cm. (*Fig.* 61) so that it should be possible to leave a generous amount of the needle protruding from the tissues when giving an inferior dental block (page 77). However, when assessing the depth of penetration the divergence of the ascending ramus upwards and its flare outwards must also be borne in mind (*Fig.* 62).

ANAESTHESIA OF THE LOWER ANTERIOR TEETH

Nerve fibrils from the teeth and supporting structures in the anterior

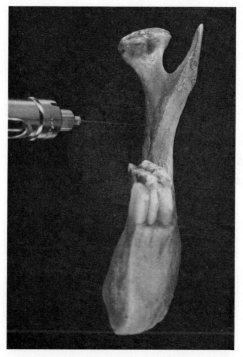

Fig. 62.—The mandible viewed from the front to emphasize the upward divergence and outward flare of the ascending ramus lateral to the arch of the lower teeth.

part of the mandible unite to form the right and left incisive nerves, which join their respective inferior dental nerves. There is considerable overlap in the midline and it is this anastomosis that renders an inferior dental block ineffective in the incisor region. Fortunately, the labial alveolar plate in this area is thinner and more porous than elsewhere (*Fig.* 63) and so it is possible to use infiltration techniques as illustrated in *Figs.* 63 and 64.

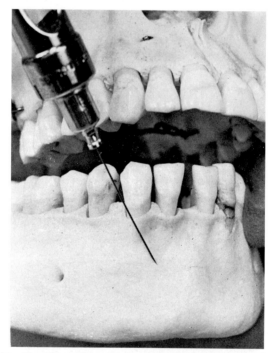

Fig. 63.—The position of the needle for infiltration of the second lower incisors.

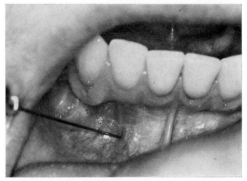

Fig. 64.—The infiltration technique is used to anaesthetize the lower incisors.

About 1 ml. of solution deposited in the labial sulcus usually suffices to produce pulpal anaesthesia but if surgery is to be undertaken up to 0·5 ml. must be injected into the lingual sulcus because anastomosis via the lingual nerve also occurs in this site.

If anaesthesia of the incisors *only* is required it is possible to use labial and lingual infiltration techniques alone.

In younger patients the use of infiltration techniques may produce satisfactory anaesthesia of the lower canine tooth, but as age advances and the bone tends to become less permeable the incidence of failure to achieve anaesthesia increases. For this reason many operators use an inferior dental injection to obtain anaesthesia of this tooth whilst others prefer to utilize a mental injection for this purpose.

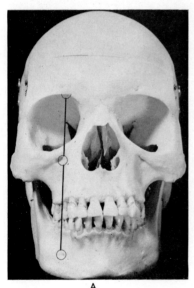 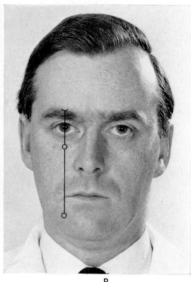

A	B

Fig. 65. An aid to the location of the infra-orbital and mental foramina. With the patient's mouth closed and his eyes looking straight ahead, a line passing vertically through the pupil of the eye will usually pass through the supra-orbital notch, infra-orbital foramen, and mental foramen. A, Skull; B, Patient.

THE MENTAL INJECTION

Anaesthetic solution deposited near the mental foramen enters the inferior dental canal to produce anaesthesia of the premolar, canine, and incisor teeth of that side. The mental foramen which is usually situated between the apices of the premolars is rarely palpable but its position may be determined by other means. For example, *Fig.* 65 illustrates how a line passing vertically downwards from the supra-orbital notch and through the infra-orbital foramen will usually cross the mental foramen when the mouth is closed.

Fig. 66 shows the mental injection being given to a patient. The left hand is used to reflect the lip in order to provide adequate visual and mechanical access. About 1 ml. of solution should be injected over the foramen. Attempts to insert the needle into the foramen may result in damage to either the nerve or blood-vessels and for this reason are contra-indicated. If surgery is to be undertaken, anaesthesia of the lingual soft tissues must also be obtained by the use of an infiltration technique. Any problem caused by overlap in the midline can be dealt with in the manner illustrated in *Figs.* 63 and 64.

When regional anaesthesia is to be supplemented by injections in the lower incisor area, it is wise to await the onset of labial symptoms before the infiltration technique is undertaken.

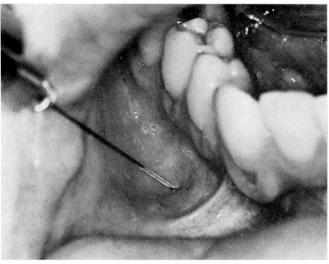

Fig. 66.—The mental nerve injection. Note that the needle is directed towards the apices of the lower premolar teeth.

ANAESTHESIA OF THE DECIDUOUS TEETH

In children multiple vascular canals perforate the labio-buccal alveolar plate. For this reason infiltration techniques are highly effective in producing anaesthesia of lower deciduous teeth. However, regional anaesthesia has the advantage of only one needle prick and the inferior dental injection, using a short needle, is preferred by many dentists and their child patients. When giving this injection it is important to remember the relationship of the inferior dental foramen to the occlusal plane (*Fig.* 60A, page 66).

Anaesthesia of the lingual nerve is invariably achieved with a successful inferior dental injection in children. However, if infiltration alone has been employed and either an extraction or the fitting of a matrix band is indicated, anaesthesia of the lingual tissues may be achieved by deposition of solution via the interproximal spaces in the manner described on page 56.

CHAPTER IX

THE DIAGNOSIS AND MANAGEMENT OF DIFFICULTIES, COMPLICATIONS, AND EMERGENCIES

THE widespread use of local anaesthesia in both dental and medical practice today is in itself a tribute to both the effectiveness and safety of the method. Nevertheless, difficulties and complications occasionally occur and it is essential that the dental surgeon should know how to minimize their incidence. However, he should never forget that any one of the many thousands of injections he gives may cause an untoward or even a dangerous reaction and must take steps to ensure that he has both the knowledge and means to diagnose and deal effectively with such a situation. In order to do this he must be familiar with the aetiology of the difficulties and complications and both he and his staff should be both proficient and practised in dealing with emergencies.

Untoward reactions of particular importance may be listed as follows:—

A. Local:—
1. Failure to obtain anaesthesia.
2. Pain during and after injection.
3. Haematoma formation at the site of injection.
4. Intra-vascular injection.
5. Blanching.
6. Trismus.
7. Facial paralysis.
8. Prolonged impairment of sensation.
9. Broken needles.
10. Infection.
11. Lip trauma.
12. Visual disturbances.

B. General:—
1. Fainting (vaso-vagal attack).
2. Drug interactions.
3. Serum hepatitis.
4. Sensitivity reactions.
5. Occupational dermatitis.
6. Cardio-respiratory emergencies.

UNTOWARD REACTIONS—LOCAL

Failure to obtain Anaesthesia.—Although the incidence of this difficulty tends to decrease as the experience and competence of the operator increases it is still probably the most common problem encountered during the use of local anaesthesia.

It may be complete or partial and every experienced dental surgeon has seen patients in whom the administration of an inferior dental block injection did not render the dentine insensitive during cavity preparation but sufficed for the extraction of an adjacent tooth. In some instances the onset of anaesthesia is merely delayed whilst in others analgesia alone is obtained when anaesthesia is desired.

Failure to secure anaesthesia is sometimes preventable for it is often due to faulty technique which results in an inadequate amount of the local anaesthetic solution being deposited in close proximity to the nerve or injection into a blood-vessel (page 73). In such cases, anaesthesia can usually be secured by repeating the injection after carefully checking the anatomical landmarks and the technique employed.

It is widely believed that a purulent response to infection is accompanied by a change in the pH of the tissues involved. In the more acid environment that ensues local anaesthetic solutions are unlikely to be effective because the agents, which are alkaloids, are not dissociated in an active state. Furthermore, injection of the solution locally involves the risk of spreading the infection beyond the defensive barriers. In these circumstances the use of a regional technique or general anaesthesia may be indicated.

Failure to achieve anaesthesia may also be due to the use of a solution after the expiration date recommended by the manufacturer. For this reason the dentist should ensure that his stock of anaesthetic cartridges is not excessive and is used in strict rotation.

Very rarely patients are seen who appear to exhibit an individual resistance to the effects of certain drugs. In such cases the use of an alternative drug of different chemical composition enables the desired result to be achieved.

Pain during and after Injection.—There can be no doubt that a considerable number of patients dread injections. Whilst in some cases this exaggerated fear is merely one aspect of the patient's attitude to life in general and dentistry in particular, it is a regrettable fact that in other cases such fears are founded on a previous painful experience. It is incumbent upon the dentist to ensure that the methods of pain control that he employs are as painless and pleasant as it is possible to make them.

The sharpness of the needle is of paramount importance and this will be ensured if only good quality disposable needles supplied by a reputable manufacturer are used. If the tissues are tensed and the sharp point of a fine gauge needle is presented at right angles to the mucosa, puncture is effected immediately. A simple experiment with two rubber balloons will convince the student that a sharp needle penetrates a tightly stretched surface much more readily than a flaccid one.

Other measures which minimize discomfort include warming the solution and injecting it slowly (pages 35 and 36).

Pain may result from the injection of either non-isotonic or contaminated solutions. The correct use of cartridges produced by a reputable manufacturer eliminates this possibility. Rarely during the administration of an inferior dental block injection the patient experiences a sharp neuralgic pain in the tissues supplied by that nerve. This symptom is an indication that the needle has penetrated the nerve sheath and it should be withdrawn. If the dentist persists with an injection in such circumstances prolonged impairment of labial sensation will result. The use of excessive force to deposit solution in resistant tissue is painful and should be avoided.

Pain from any of the causes described above may persist after the effect of the anaesthetic has disappeared. Other causes of after-pain or discomfort include infection (page 77), trismus (page 74), and haematoma formation.

Haematoma Formation.—Due to the highly vascular nature of the oral soft tissues it is inevitable that the point of a needle enters a blood-vessel on occasions. Different investigators using aspiration techniques have stated that the incidence of this mishap varies between 2 and 11 per cent. It is least common when infiltration techniques are used and occurs most frequently when posterior superior dental blocks are given. This is due to the structure and variable position of the pterygoid venous plexus. Less frequently, a vessel may be trapped against bone and punctured by the needle during the administration of either an inferior dental or an infra-orbital injection.

The mishap is followed by bleeding into the tissues with haematoma formation and predisposes to the risk of intra-vascular injection (*see below*). Bleeding from the pterygoid venous plexus produces a rapid and dramatic swelling of the cheek which is followed by discoloration of the overlying skin due to breakdown of blood pigments within 24–28 hours.

Bleeding from the infra-orbital venous plexus produces a similar sequence of events and a 'black eye'. The patient should be told that the bleeding will stop spontaneously, that these swellings usually disperse within 24–48 hours, and that the discoloration will disappear in a manner similar to a bruise. Many patients experience discomfort due to the irritant effects of blood in tissue spaces and should be warned accordingly.

Bleeding into the pterygo-mandibular space as the result of an inferior dental injection is usually not apparent immediately and the patient frequently returns a day or two later complaining of trismus (page 74).

If the dentist thinks that the haematoma is likely to become infected antibiotic therapy must be instituted promptly regardless of the site of the clot which, being avascular, forms an ideal nidus for the proliferation of bacteria. The patient should also be recalled for review within 24 hours and subsequently if necessary.

Intra-vascular Injection.—Penetration of a blood-vessel can only be detected promptly if the technique of aspiration has been employed (page 23). If, during aspiration, blood is seen to pass into the solution a vessel has been entered and the needle must be withdrawn immediately and re-inserted in a slightly different position.

If an aspirating syringe is not used the incidence of intra-vascular injections is increased. This risk will be reduced but not eliminated if, when bone is contacted, the needle is withdrawn slightly prior to the deposition of solution.

The intra-vascular injection of any drug increases its possible toxic effects. Although in the case of local anaesthetic solutions reactions may be produced by either the anaesthetic agent or the vasoconstrictor or both, in practice it is virtually impossible to determine the substance responsible. Frequently, the patient feels faint, has a pale clammy skin, and rapid pulse (tachycardia). The onset of these manifestations is an indication to abandon the injection and adopt the procedure detailed on page 79. Unless measures are taken promptly temporary loss of consciousness may ensue.

Blanching.—Blanching at the site of injection or elsewhere may be caused by an injection. The former is due to a combination of increased tissue tension due to the deposition of fluid and the local effect of the vaso-constrictor. Blanching at a site remote from that of the injection may be due either to intra-vascular injection or to interference with the autonomic nerve-supply of the blood-vessels.

The ischaemia is transitory and may last from thirty seconds to thirty minutes. No treatment other than reassurance is required. Careful injection technique including either aspiration prior to injection or slight withdrawal of the needle before injecting should reduce the incidence of this complication.

Trismus.—Trismus may be defined as difficulty in opening the jaws due to muscle spasm. Trismus can be caused by injection into the medial pterygoid muscle, when damage to blood-vessels may result in a haematoma or infection. Whilst it is usually realized that inflammation will cause an adjacent muscle to go into spasm it is often not appreciated that blood within tissue spaces is very irritant and may produce a similar effect.

The onset of trismus is often some time after the injection and completion of the dental procedure. If it is due to infection, the patient may have a rise in temperature and complain of both pain and feeling unwell. In such circumstances any pus present must be drained and antibiotic therapy instituted. When any infection has been controlled the symptoms of trismus may be alleviated by the use of hot saline mouth baths and short wave diathermy.

Facial Paralysis.—Paralysis of the facial muscles on one side is an uncommon complication of an inferior dental injection and may be either partial or complete depending upon which branches of the nerve are affected.

This complication arises if the tip of the needle is inserted too far back and behind the ascending ramus. The solution is then deposited in the substance of the parotid gland where it anaesthetizes the branches of the facial nerve causing paralysis of the muscles they supply (*Fig.* 67). Since the parotid gland is enveloped by a fascial sheath there is also a failure to obtain anaesthesia of the inferior dental nerve.

The patient afflicted with this alarming and unsightly complication must be reassured that normal function and appearance will return as soon as the effects of the local anaesthetic agent wear off. Nevertheless, if the nerve-supply to the eyelids has been affected it is a wise precaution to close the lids and apply a protective pad or eye-shade.

Prolonged Impairment of Sensation.—Prolonged impairment of sensation following the use of local anaesthesia is due to nerve damage. This may be caused by direct trauma from the bevel of the needle or the injection of a solution contaminated with a neurotoxic substance such as alcohol (page 16). The risk of injecting the wrong solution by mistake may be eliminated completely by using the clearly labelled cartridges supplied by reputable manufacturers.

Haemorrhage and infection in close proximity to a nerve may also produce prolonged impairment of sensation. Surgery or infection related to lower molar and premolar roots sometimes causes impairment of sensation in the lower lip. In those cases due to infection any pus present must be drained and antibiotic therapy instituted promptly. In other circumstances

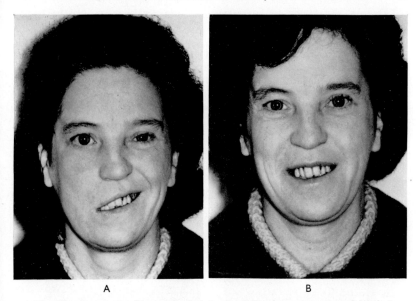

Fig. 67.—A patient with a right facial palsy following an unsuccessful inferior dental injection. A, Attempts to smile produce only a unilateral effect due to paralysis of the facial muscles. B, Three hours later complete recovery has occurred.

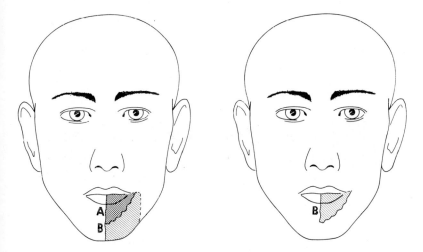

Fig. 68.—An example of a method of recording the extent of impaired sensation of the mental nerve, Left, an area of anaesthesia (A) and an area of paraesthesia (B). Right, the record of improvement over a period of about 6 weeks. The area of paraesthesia has returned to normal and the area of anaesthesia has progressed to paraesthesia.

the degree and extent of anaesthesia or paraesthesia should be tested. Reactions to pin-pricks and the passing of cotton-wool wisps over the skin may be used for this purpose, but the patient's eyes must be closed to avoid false impressions of sensation. The affected areas should then be recorded (*Fig.* 68) and the patient seen at regular intervals so that the speed and degree of recovery of sensation may be determined. Definite signs and symptoms of recovery are usually apparent within 3 months. Should the operator suspect that no improvement is taking place he should refer the patient for a specialist opinion.

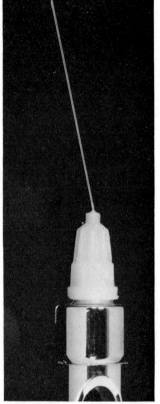
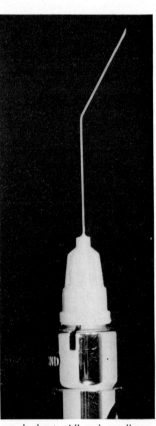

Fig. 69.—Common sites at which a needle may be bent. All such needles *must* be discarded.

Broken Needles.—The introduction of high quality stainless-steel needles which are packaged, pre-sterilized, and disposable has reduced greatly the incidence of this complication. Prior to the introduction of disposable needles, some dental surgeons kept fine hypodermic needles in a chemical disinfectant solution. This not only failed to produce sterilization, but corroded the metal and predisposed to breakage. If a needle other than the disposable type has to be used it should be sterilized (page 21) immediately before use and discarded on completion of the procedure.

The needle must be kept straight during its passage through the tissues. If undue resistance is encountered force must not be applied to overcome it nor should the direction of the needle be changed without withdrawing it from the tissues. In this way bending of the needle should be avoided. However, should it occur, the bent needle must be discarded since attempts to straighten it invariably cause weakening and increase the risk of fracture during subsequent use (*Fig.* 69).

When needles fracture they usually do so at the hub. For this reason a needle should never be embedded completely within the tissues but at least 5 mm. must project from the mucosal surface. Should fracture occur, the tissues must be kept under continuous pressure whilst the protruding end is grasped with either pliers or artery forceps and the broken fragment withdrawn (page 35).

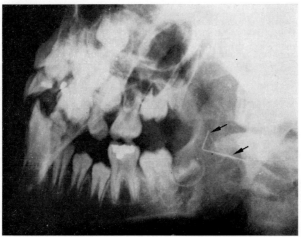

Fig. 70.—Lateral oblique radiograph of a 9-year-old girl in which a needle fragment (arrowed) is clearly demonstrated. (*Courtesy of Mr. J. W. Frame.*)

If a fragment of a needle is retained within the tissues the patient should be informed and the situation explained to him. No attempt should be made to remove it at this stage but radiographs should be taken to confirm its presence and position (*Fig.* 70). Careful notes of the incident should be made which include details of the precise sequence of events. The broken portion of the needle should be removed from the syringe and kept in a safe place because metallurgical investigation may be required at a later date (*Fig.* 71). The patient should be referred to a consultant dental surgeon with a letter requesting his opinion, advice, and treatment as required. It is a wise precaution at this stage to send full details of the incident to the professional defence organization to which the dentist belongs.

Infection.—Infection is a comparatively rare complication of injection.

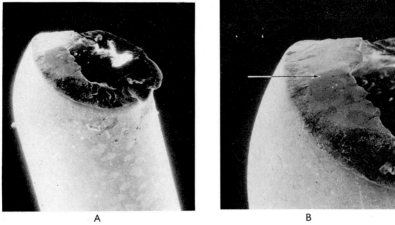

A   B

Fig. 71.—An example of a broken hypodermic needle which has been subjected to metallurgical investigation. A, The fracture line and lumen of the needle; B, Higher magnification of part of the fracture line showing 'smoothing' of the irregular surface suggesting a crack at this site before the needle was used on a patient. (*Courtesy of the Medical Defence Union.*)

The use of pre-sterilized equipment and aseptic technique virtually eliminates the chances of organisms being introduced into the tissues at the time of injection. Nevertheless, on occasions infection of a tissue space such as the pterygo-mandibular space may occur. It is wise to refer such patients for specialist opinion and treatment.

Lip Trauma.—Children who have had an inferior dental injection should

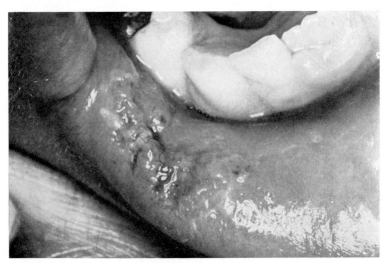

Fig. 72.—An example of ulceration of the lower lip in a child who bit it after receiving an inferior dental injection. (*Courtesy of Mr. M. A. Young.*)

be warned that it is possible to chew the anaesthetized part of the lip and so produce a very sore ulcer (*Fig.* 72). In spite of this warning the complication can occur but fortunately such lesions heal rapidly with minimal scarring.

Adults given an inferior dental injection for the first time should be warned of the risk of thermal damage to the lip from either hot drinks or cigarette smoking.

Visual Disturbances.—On very rare occasions patients may complain of unilateral or bilateral disturbance of vision. This may take the form of squints or double vision and even transient blindness has been reported. An adequate explanation of these phenomena is difficult to find but it seems possible that vascular spasm or accidental intra-arterial injection is the most likely cause. In such cases an unusual vascular distribution can be assumed and the patient reassured that normal vision will be restored within about 30 minutes.

Some maxillary injections may result in solution infiltrating the orbit to anaesthetize the motor muscles of the eye. The resulting disturbance of vision will return to normal as the solution is dispersed—usually within about 3 hours.

UNTOWARD REACTIONS—GENERAL

Fainting (Vaso-vagal Attack).—Collapse in the dental chair may occur suddenly and may or may not be accompanied by loss of consciousness. In most instances these episodes are vaso-vagal attacks or 'faints' and spontaneous recovery is usual. The patient often complains of feeling dizzy, weak, and nauseated, and the skin is pale, cold, and clammy. First aid treatment should be instituted at once and at no time should such a patient be left unattended. The head should be lowered by quickly adjusting the back of the chair so that the patient assumes the supine position with the legs elevated. Any tight collar or belt should be loosened and a cold wet swab applied to the brow. Respiration may be stimulated by holding smelling salts under the nose. Spontaneous recovery is usual and it is often possible to complete the treatment at the same visit.

A woman in the last 3 months of pregnancy should not be placed in the supine position because the gravid uterus may press on the inferior vena cava and produce the 'supine hypotensive syndrome' in addition to respiratory embarrassment. When such a patient faints she should be laid on her side, care being taken to maintain the airway. Patients exhibiting acute respiratory distress, such as occurs in bronchial asthma or pulmonary oedema, should never be laid flat but should sit forward with their arms supported on the bracket table.

Under no circumstances must fluids be given by mouth until the patient is conscious. When consciousness returns a glucose drink may be given if the patient has missed a meal before being treated under local anaesthesia. Alternatively Sp. Ammon. Aromat. B.P.C. (Sal volatile) 3·6 ml. in at least one-third of a tumblerful of water may be administered, but this does have an objectionable taste.

If signs of recovery are not apparent within 30–45 seconds of first aid measures being instituted, the collapse is probably not of vaso-vagal origin. The airway must be maintained, oxygen administered, and medical aid summoned. Careful note should be taken of both the type and rate of respiration and the rate, volume, and character of the pulse. The further management of this emergency and other causes of collapse are discussed on pages 83 and 87.

Patients occasionally present with a history of repeated fainting when local anaesthetic solutions are administered to them. They should be treated in the supine position soon after they have eaten a meal and are often helped by premedication (page 31). Even when these precautions have been taken, cases occur in which it is necessary to employ general anaesthesia.

Drug Interactions.—An assessment of the general condition of any patient requiring local anaesthesia must be an invariable routine and it is also important to make inquiries about current drug therapy because some drugs prescribed for the treatment of systemic disease may interact with those included in a local anaesthetic solution. Many such patients are unaware of the name or nature of medicines they are taking. For this reason if doubt exists the dentist should contact the doctor concerned before proceeding with dental treatment to ascertain details of the medication. At the same time he should also receive guidance concerning the severity of the systemic condition and its relationship to dental treatment.

Table IV.—Some Tricyclic Anti-depressive Drugs

Official Name	Proprietary Names
Amitriptyline	Amizol, Domical, Larozyl (Sweden), Limbitrol (also contains chlordiazepoxide), Saroten, Triptafen, and Tryptizol
Clomipramine	Anafranil
Desipramine	Pertofran
Imipramine	Berkomine, Tofranil, Praminil, Norpramine, Impril (Canada), Imiprin (Australia), and Iramil
Nortriptyline	Allegron, Aventyl; Motipress and Motival are compound preparations of nortriptyline and fluphenazine
Opipramol	Insidon
Protriptyline	Concordin
Trimipramine	Surmontil

(*From 'The Extraction of Teeth', 2nd Ed. revised reprint, by Geoffrey L. Howe, Bristol, Wright, 1980*).

In recent years the treatment of depressive illness has been revolutionized by the introduction of the monoamine oxidase inhibitor and tricyclic drugs. When the former were first introduced it was thought that they would potentiate the action of adrenaline or noradrenaline to provoke a dangerous rise in blood-pressure. In the light of experience it is now accepted that the small amounts of amine vasoconstrictors contained in local anaesthetic solutions do not constitute any danger to dental patients taking this type of drug.

Greater caution must be exercised if local anaesthesia is for patients taking any of the tricyclic group of anti-depressive drugs (*Table IV*), some of which are also used to treat nocturnal enuresis in children. It has been demonstrated that the effects of noradrenaline are potentiated significantly by drugs of the tricyclic group and the effects of adrenaline to a lesser extent. These vasoconstrictors should not be injected in patients taking tricyclic anti-depressive drugs because of the risk of producing hypertension or cardiac arrhythmia. Solutions that do not contain either adrenaline or noradrenaline (*Table I*, page 14), or a prilocaine preparation containing felypressin, a non-amine vasoconstrictor (Citanest with Octapressin), should be used under these circumstances.

A profound hypertensive reaction is characterized by the sudden onset of a severe headache. Whilst this phenomenon is usually transient, it may be complicated by either intra-cranial haemorrhage or acute heart failure. These complications may be avoided by the intramuscular or intravenous injection of 5 mg. phentolamine (Rogitine), but as such treatment may produce a labile blood-pressure it is best carried out by experts with the aid of electronic monitoring equipment. For this reason any patient exhibiting such a reaction should be transferred to hospital without delay.

Occasionally a dentist performing surgery under general anaesthesia may wish to use a solution containing a vasoconstrictor in order to reduce the vascularity of the operative site. If so, he should always consult the anaesthetist prior to the induction of anaesthesia, for adrenaline or noradrenaline may provoke cardiac arrhythmia when used in conjunction with such agents as halothane, ethyl chloride, trichlorethylene, and cyclopropane. There is no evidence that felypressin produces a similar complication, so that prilocaine with felypressin may be used safely under these circumstances although it is less effective.

Although procaine is now seldom employed in dentistry it should be noted that this local anaesthetic agent should not be used in patients receiving sulphonamides for the treatment of systemic disease. As this group of anti-bacterial drugs contain the same para-amino benzoic acid ring as procaine, it is theoretically possible that they could partially neutralize the effects of each other if administered concurrently. Although this phenomenon has never been proved clinically, the combination is better avoided. Any patient who gives a history of hypersensitivity to sulphonamides should not receive a local anaesthetic agent containing the para-amino benzoic acid ring (*Table I*, page 14).

Serum Hepatitis.—The causative agent of this very serious disease is the Hepatitis B associated antigen (HBsAg) which has also been called 'Virus B' and 'Australian antigen'. Some healthy people harbour this antigen in their blood for prolonged periods, perhaps even indefinitely, without exhibiting any clinical symptoms of serum hepatitis. However, if the antigen is transmitted from such individuals to one who is susceptible to it the full manifestations of serum hepatitis may be produced. Patients contracting the disease as a result of treatment by their dentists are rarely seen by them because the incubation period may be as long as 160 days. By this time the patient does not associate his condition with dental treatment and consults his doctor. In dental practice the risk of cross-infection is greatest if inadequately sterilized syringes and needles are used. A Medical Research Council report published as long ago as 1962 contained a reference to the admission to one hospital during a 2-year period of 15 cases, 3 of which were fatal, following dental procedures. The high risk of transmission of this dangerous disease during dental procedures is the reason why a hypodermic needle should never be used on more than one patient (page 28). The high risk of transmission of this dangerous disease during dental injections was emphasized in the report of the Expert Group on Hepatitis in Dentistry (1979) which recommended that it must be universal practice to use a fresh cartridge and new disposable needle for each patient.

Sensitivity Reactions.—Hypersensitivity reactions to local anaesthetic agents may vary in degree from local oedematous swelling or urticaria at the site of injection to a profound and dangerous anaphylactic reaction which can prove fatal if not treated promptly. This phenomenon is due to a pathological response of the tissues of sensitized individuals to certain substances known as 'allergens'. Any local anaesthetic agent may evoke such a response. Although patients afflicted with allergic diseases such as bronchial asthma are especially liable to be hypersensitive to these drugs, otherwise healthy 'normal' people may also react abnormally on rare occasions.

Local reactions are seen more frequently than systemic reactions and usually resolve without active treatment. Should they fail to do so the administration of an anti-histaminic drug such as chlorpheniramine maleate (Piriton) 4 mg. tablets three times a day for a maximum of 3 days usually effects a cure.

Anaphylaxis is characterized by a profound fall in blood-pressure, loss of consciousness, respiratory embarrassment, facial and laryngeal oedema, and urticaria. Unless treatment is instituted immediately the condition may progress to a fatal termination. Treatment consists of the slow intravenous injection of hydrocortisone hemisuccinate sodium 100 mg. in 2 ml. More severe allergic reactions can be relieved by the intramuscular injection of 1 ml. of 0·1 per cent (1 in 1000) adrenaline solution repeated every 5 minutes until the symptoms begin to subside or until the maximum dose of 5 ml. has been given. Such a heavy dosage of adrenaline is not without dangers for it can cause acute cardiac failure but in the presence of severe anaphylactic shock this risk must be accepted if the patient is to survive.

Some vials of 1 in 1000 adrenaline solution together with a 2 ml. disposable syringe should always be conveniently at hand when injections are given, for although they will be required only on very rare occasions, speed is essential when they are needed if the patient's life is to be saved. Adrenaline should be stored in a cool dark place and only clear colourless solutions should be used. The drug deteriorates rapidly in daylight to form a brownish pinkish solution.

The potentially serious nature of hypersensitivity reactions makes it essential that all patients for whom a drug is prescribed should be carefully and thoroughly questioned concerning any previous experiences with the drug. If reasonable grounds emerge for the operator to suspect allergy, the patient should be referred for sensitivity tests. These may consist of injecting very small quantities of local anaesthetic and control solutions intradermally at a suitable skin site and observing any idiosyncratic reaction. Topical application of local anaesthetic solution in one nostril is another commonly used test. However, the interpretation of reactions can present difficulties and is best left to expert allergists. Regardless of whether or not allergy is confirmed, it is good practice, whenever a patient gives any history of unconfirmed reactions to local anaesthesia, to utilize another local anaesthetic agent of different chemical structure (*Table I*, page 14) and to seek specialist advice on this choice if it is practicable to do so.

Occupational Dermatitis.—When procaine was the local anaesthetic of choice it was not uncommon for dentists and dental nurses to acquire a sensitivity to it. The resulting condition was known as 'Novocain' dermatitis and was characterized by painful cracking and fissuring of the skin which was especially marked around the nails and between the fingers. The condition was resistant to treatment and those afflicted were compelled to wear rubber gloves whilst working, in an attempt to avoid contact with procaine.

The widespread use in modern practice of local anaesthetic agents of an entirely different composition, such as lignocaine, which is an anilide derivative, has made occupational dermatitis a rarity in dentists and dental nurses. However, it is still seen occasionally and is usually due to the use of certain topical anaesthetic preparations which contain para-aminobenzoic-acid derivatives, such as benzocaine. If the dentist suspects that he may be developing such an incapacitating allergy he should cease to use the preparation concerned and seek the opinion and advice of a dermatologist.

Cardio-respiratory Emergencies.—The chances of respiratory failure or cardiac arrest being caused directly by the injection of local anaesthetic solution are remote. Nevertheless, every dental surgeon must be capable of dealing with such emergencies should they occur for any reason. It is important to appreciate that the two conditions are inter-related because if either goes undetected and untreated it will progress rapidly to the other. If, therefore, a patient stops breathing it is essential to check the carotid pulse and look at the pupils of the eyes. Absence of this pulse and dilatation of the pupils are two signs that indicate that cardiac arrest may be the cause of the respiratory failure. For purposes of description it is convenient to describe the two conditions as separate entities.

Respiratory Arrest.—Complete cessation of breathing is usually preceded by depression of both the rate and depth of respiration and is best assessed in general dental practice by observing the excursions of the chest. If depression is recognized but respiration is still present pure oxygen should be administered using a full face mask. This procedure will usually affect recovery within 4 to 5 minutes.

If breathing has stopped the patient must be laid flat on the floor with his head turned to one side whilst his airway is cleared by the removal of any foreign material either manually or by suction apparatus. Dentures or orthodontic appliances should also be removed and the neck extended fully by pulling the mandible upwards and forwards. The face is turned upwards to facilitate the insertion of an airway (*Fig.* 73) and ventilation of the lungs is started without delay. A manual pulmonary resuscitator (*Fig.* 74) may be used for this purpose or mouth-to-mouth resuscitation (*Fig.* 75) may be employed if such apparatus is not available. In either case the period of inflation should be 1·0–1·5 seconds and a period of about 2 seconds then allowed for the patient to exhale passively. Such a procedure will achieve the normal respiratory rate of 15–20 breaths per minute. If recovery is not apparent within 20 minutes the patient should be transferred to hospital by ambulance and the ventilation continued by the dentist throughout the journey. This responsibility must not be delegated to ambulance attendants.

Cardiac Arrest.—Signs of cardiovascular failure are invariably apparent before cardiac arrest occurs. The skin, especially of the face, may be pale and sweating evident. Any patient showing early signs of cardiovascular failure must immediately be laid flat, with the head to one side, to counter the effects of the semi-erect posture and reduce the gravitational factors due to the difference in height between the heart and the brain. After the release of tight clothing the legs should be raised to encourage the flow of

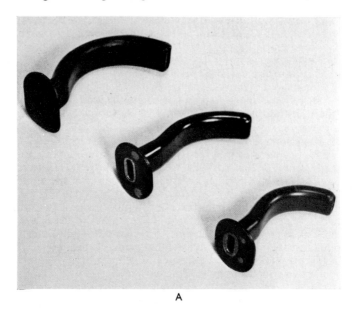

A

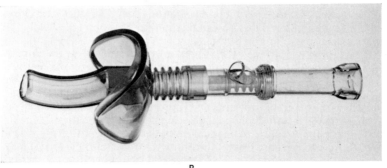

B

Fig. 73.—A, Three different sizes of Guedel airways which are inserted behind the tongue and used in conjunction with an oxygen mask or a manual resuscitator. B, A Brook airway which has a removable extension tube with non-return valve for oral ventilation.

venous blood to the heart thus improving cardiac output. If immediate improvement is not apparent oxygen should be administered as described previously and in most cases spontaneous recovery will occur.

However, in a small number of patients the condition may progress to cardiac arrest. This diagnosis must be made immediately for unless the circulation can be restored and maintained within about 3 minutes irreversible brain damage may occur due to cerebral anoxia. Two features confirm that cardiac arrest has occurred, namely, the absence of a carotid pulse and failure of the dilating pupil to respond to light. Under these circumstances external cardiac massage must be instituted immediately. Time should not be wasted seeking the apical cardiac impulse since this is very difficult to detect under these circumstances. The heart will often

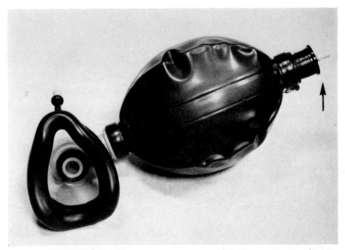

Fig. 74.—An Ambu manual resuscitator to which an oxygen supply may be attached where indicated by the arrow if required.

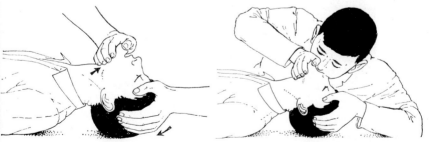

Fig. 75.—Mouth-to-mouth resuscitation. A, Extending the head to clear the airway. B, Technique of artificial respiration. If the external nares cannot be covered by the operator's mouth they must be compressed between his finger and thumb. (*Figs.* 74 *and* 75 *from 'The Extraction of Teeth', 2nd Ed., by Geoffrey L. Howe, Bristol, Wright,* 1970.)

start beating again if the sternum is struck sharply but patients who do not respond to this manœuvre must be placed flat on the floor to facilitate cardiac massage. Since manual ventilation must be combined with this treatment a position near the suction apparatus and oxygen supply should be selected.

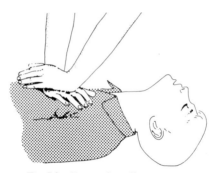

Fig. 76.—External cardiac massage.

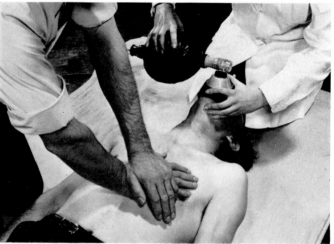

Fig. 77.—External cardiac massage being applied and synchronized with ventilation of the lungs by means of a manual resuscitator.

External cardiac massage is performed by the dentist kneeling on one side of the trunk. The heel of one hand is placed over the lower third of the sternum. If the fingers of this hand point towards the shoulder the risk of undue pressure on internal organs will be reduced. The flat of the other hand is then placed on top of it and pressure applied vertically downwards once every second. This firm but steady pressure should depress the sternum about 4–5 cm. in an average adult thereby compressing the heart against the vertebral column. At the end of each compressive movement the hands are lifted to allow full recoil and expansion of the chest. This is the moment at which manual ventilation of the lungs is most effective and efforts should be made to achieve this synchronization (*Fig.* 77). When no assistance is available the dental surgeon should perform respiratory and cardiac resuscitation alternatively for periods of 20 seconds. Prolonged resuscitation is an exhausting procedure and although theoretically it should be continued until the patient's colour improves, his pupils contract, and respiration and heart-beats are restored, an unassisted operator can only maintain resuscitation for a limited period. This period can be prolonged greatly if assistance is available and the individuals participating in the resuscitation of the patient take turns at pulmonary inflation and cardiac massage alternately.

In children under the age of about 10 years a more gentle approach is necessary and adequate compression of the sternum of 3–4 cm. may be achieved with one hand. Artificial ventilation of the lungs should also be less vigorous in children than in adults.

Drugs in the management of cardio-respiratory emergencies are best reserved for the use of experts who invariably prefer to monitor their effects with specialized equipment. For this reason the average dental practitioner should confine his treatment to the 'first aid' measures described and summon assistance when a serious cardio-respiratory crisis becomes apparent. He should be fortified by the knowledge that a calm and sensible application of simple mechanical principles will sustain his patient in the majority of the rare emergencies of this nature which occur in a dental surgery.

PRECAUTIONARY MEASURES

It is the duty of the dental surgeon to make every endeavour to avoid complications and to prevent emergencies from arising. Although it is not possible to prevent their occurrence, both their incidence and their effects can be reduced by the exercise of care and skill. Complications can only be diagnosed and emergencies dealt with promptly and effectively if the possibility of their occurrence has been anticipated. All too often a serious incident has been required to stimulate a practitioner into carrying out a critical survey of the emergency arrangements in his practice.

As fainting occurs more frequently when the temperature and relative humidity are high, the surgery should be kept cool and well ventilated. It has been shown that dental patients, especially men under 35 years of age, with a history of fainting in the dental surgery on previous occasions, are more likely to faint than others. Special efforts should be made to reassure such a patient. He must be carefully observed and at the first sign of pallor he should be laid flat, for in this position he is less likely to lose consciousness. In many instances treatment can be carried out in the supine position.

The dental surgeon should use a dental chair, the design of which permits the patient to be placed quickly upon his back with his legs higher than his head in an emergency. Otherwise an unconscious patient will have to be lifted out of the chair and on to the floor. Little purpose will be served by this exhausting manœuvre if there is insufficient free space available for the patient to be laid down and resuscitated. As it may be necessary to remove blood, mucus, or vomit from the air passages, an efficient aspiration apparatus should be kept readily available in the surgery. A supply of oxygen and either a modern anaesthetic machine or a manual resuscitator (e.g., Ambu (*Fig.* 74), Air Viva, or Laerdal) with which a patient's lungs can be inflated with either air or preferably oxygen should also be near at hand. It is as useless to have oxygen available for use when the tubing is too short to allow the mask to be applied to the face of a supine patient as to know which drug should be given if it, and the apparatus and expertise required to administer it, are not readily available.

Times of stress and crisis are ill-suited for either the acquisition of new clinical skills or the institution of a search in the telephone directory for the numbers of doctors or hospitals. For these reasons every dental surgeon should try to foresee possible emergencies and prepare for them. He should instruct each member of his staff in the role that he or she will play when a crisis occurs and should hold regular practices and checks on his emergency equipment and arrangements. If only one emergency occurs during a lifetime of practice and the life of the patient concerned is preserved as a result of his precautionary measures, the wisdom and foresight of the dentist will have been amply rewarded.

INDEX